DIET ANALYSIS
Quick Reference

by
Gordon M. Wardlaw, Ph.D., R.D., L.D.
Paul M. Insel, Ph.D.

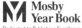

Mosby
Year Book
Dedicated to Publishing Excellence

Copyright © 1992 by Mosby-Year Book, Inc.
11830 Westline Industrial Drive
St. Louis, MO 63146

Printed in the United States of America

PREFACE

The 1988 Surgeon General's Report warns us that "for the two out of three adult Americans who do not smoke or drink excessively, one personal choice seems to influence long-term health prospects more than any other: what we eat." We have developed a handy quick reference to help you learn more about what you eat and improve your lifetime health. In this pocket-sized reference lies the information you need to accurately track your nutrient intake. The food composition tables list kcalories, fat, carbohydrate, protein, dietary fiber, saturated fat, and cholesterol content for nearly 900 foods. A separate fast food table provides the same information for popular foods at ten leading fast food restaurants in the U.S. Nutrition experts tell us to eat more carbohydrate and dietary fiber while eating less fat, saturated fat, and cholesterol. This quick reference will help you do just that.

Watching food intake is just the beginning of a healthy approach to life. Increasing energy (i.e. kcalorie) expenditure in the form of daily activity and more formal physical activities, such as tennis and jogging, is a key part of a complete health promotion plan. In this guide, we provide an energy cost chart that will aid you in determining energy use during various activities. In addition, we provide diet forms that allow you to track your energy output. By comparing your energy intake with your energy output you can determine if you are in kcalorie balance—intake equaling output. This balance is key to healthful living and is very important for each one of us.

Knowledge is power. This quick reference gives you a powerful tool for learning more about you eat, and whether it is in overall balance with your energy needs. Carry this handy reference with you and learn more about healthful living.

Gordon M. Wardlaw, Ph.D., R.D., L.D.
Paul M. Insel, Ph.D.

CONTENTS

Food Composition Table 1

Fast Food Table 39

Energy Cost of Various Activities 50

Food Record Forms 54

FOOD COMPOSITION TABLES

Food Name

BABY FOODS

Food Name	Serving	KCAL Kc	PROT Gm	CARB Gm	FAT Gm	CHOL Mg	SAFA Gm	FIBD Gm
Baby-carrots	ounce	8	0.2	1.7	0	0	0	0.7
Baby-teething biscuits	item	43	1.2	8.4	0.5	0	-	0.1
Baby-mixed cereal/milk	ounce	32	1.3	4.5	1	0	-	0.25
Baby-oatmeal cereal/milk	ounce	33	1.4	4.3	1.2	0	-	0.7
Baby-rice cereal/milk	ounce	33	1.1	4.7	1	0	-	0.25
Baby-beef lasagna	ounce	22	1.2	2.8	0.6	-	-	0.1
Baby-beef stew	ounce	14	1.4	1.5	0.3	3.55	0.16	0.34
Baby-mixed vegetables	ounce	11	0.3	2.7	0.028	0	0	0.25
Baby-turkey & rice	ounce	14	0.5	2.1	0.4	2.84	0.12	0
Baby-veal & vegetables	ounce	20	1.7	1.7	0.8	-	-	0.1
Baby-apple blueberry	ounce	17	0.1	4.6	0.1	0	0.	0.1
Baby-applesauce	ounce	12	0.1	3.1	0.1	0	0.	0.7
Baby-peaches	ounce	20	0.1	5.4	0	0	0	0.7
Baby-pears	ounce	12	0.1	3.1	0	0	0	0.55
Baby-apple juice	fl oz	14	0	3.6	0	0	0	0.25
Baby-apple peach juice	fl oz	13	0	3.2	0	0	0	0.25
Baby-orange juice	fl oz	14	0.2	3.2	0.1	0	0	0.25
Baby-beef	ounce	30	3.9	0	1.5	-	0.73	0
Baby-chicken	ounce	37	3.9	0	2.2	-	0.58	0
Baby-egg yolks	serving	58	2.8	0.3	4.9	223	1.47	0
Baby-ham	ounce	32	3.9	0	1.6	-	0.55	0
Baby-lamb	ounce	29	4	0	1.3	0	0.66	0
Baby-liver	ounce	29	4.1	0.4	1.1	52	0.39	0
Baby-pork	ounce	35	4	0	2	-	0.68	0

2

Food Name	Serving	KCAL Kc	PROT Gm	CARB Gm	FAT Gm	CHOL Mg	SAFA Gm	FIBD Gm
Baby-turkey	ounce	32	4	0	1.7	-	0.54	0
Baby-beans-green	ounce	7	0.4	1.7	0	0	0	0.39
Baby-cookie-arrowroot	item	24	0.4	4.3	0.9	0	0.2	0.1
Baby-garden vegetables	ounce	11	0.7	1.9	0.1	0	0	0.7
Baby-peas	ounce	11	1	2.3	0.1	0	0	0.7
Baby-squash	ounce	7	0.2	1.6	0.1	0	0	0.7
Baby-sweet potatoes	ounce	16	0.3	3.7	0	0	0	0.7
Baby-pretzels	item	24	0.7	4.9	0.1	0	0	0
Baby-Zwieback	piece	30	0.7	5.2	0.7	1.46	0.28	0
Baby-cereal & egg yolks	ounce	15	0.5	2	0.5	18	0.17	0
Baby-apple betty	ounce	20	0.1	5.6	0	-	0	0.1
Baby-beef & egg noodles	ounce	15	0.6	2	0.5	-	-	0.1
Baby-beans-green-buttered	ounce	9	0.3	1.9	0.2	-	-	0.7
Baby-beets	ounce	10	0.4	2.2	0	0	0	0.4
Baby-corn-creamed	ounce	16	0.4	4	0.1	0	0	0.9
Baby-peas-creamed	ounce	15	0.6	2.5	0.5	0	0	0.7
Baby-spinach-creamed	ounce	11	0.7	1.6	0.4	0	-	1.12
BEVERAGES								
Carn inst break-choc-env	item	130	7	23	1	-	-	-
Choc bev drink-no milk-dry	ounce	99.1	0.937	25.6	0.88	0	0.521	-
Beer-regular	fl oz	12.2	0.089	1.1	0	0	0	0.07
Whis/gin/rum/Vod-80 proof	fl oz	64	0	0	0	0	0	0
Whis/gin/rum/Vod-86 proof	fl oz	69.5	0	0.028	0	0	0	0
Whis/gin/rum/Vod-90 proof	fl oz	72.9	0	0	0	0	0	0

Food Name	Serving	KCAL Kc	PROT Gm	CARB Gm	FAT Gm	CHOL Mg	SAFA Gm	FIBD Gm
Wine-dessert	fl oz	45.9	0.06	3.54	0	0	0	0
Wine-red-table	fl oz	21	0.059	0.502	0	0	0	0
Club soda	fl oz	0	0	0	0	0	0	0
Coffee-brewed	fl oz	0.592	0.03	0.118	0	0	0.001	0
Coffee-instant-prepared	cup	4.78	0.239	0.956	0	0	0.005	0
Tea-brewed	fl oz	0.296	0	0.089	0	0	0.001	0
Tea-instant-prep-unsweet	cup	2.37	0.259	0.474	0	0	0	0
Tea-instant-prep-sweetened	cup	88.1		22.1	0	0	0.008	0
Cordials/liqueur-54 proof	fl oz	97	-	11.5	0	0	0	0
Brandy-cognac-pony	item	73	-	-	0	0	0	0
Cider-fermented	fl oz	11.8	-	0.3	0	0	0	0
Whis/gin/rum vod-94 proof	fl oz	76.5	0	0	0	0	0	0
Whis/gin/rum vod-100 proof	fl oz	82	0	0	0	0	0	0
Champagne-domestic-glass	item	84	0.2	3	0	0	0	0
Wine-vermouth-dry-glass	item	105	0	1	0	0	0	0
Wine-vermouth-sweet-glass	item	167	0	12	0	0	0	0
Beer-light	fl oz	8.26	0.059	0.384	0	0	0	0
Hot cocoa-prep/milk-home	cup	218	9.1	25.8	9.05	33.3	5.61	3
Cream soda	fl oz	15.8	0	4.1	0	0	0	0
Perrier-mineral water	cup	0	0	0	0	0	0	0
Ovaltine-choc-prep/milk	cup	227	9.53	29.2	8.79	-	-	-
Coffee substitute-prepared	fl oz	1.52	0.03	0.303	0.028	0	0.002	0
Postum-inst grain bev-dry	ounce	103	1.93	24.1	0	0	0	0
Tang-inst drink-orange-dry	ounce	104	0	26.1	0	0	0	-
Wine-white-table	fl oz	20.1	0.03	0.236	0	0	0	0
Fruit punch drink-can	fl oz	14.6	0	3.69	0	0	0.001	0

Food Name	Serving	KCAL Kc	PROT Gm	CARB Gm	FAT Gm	CHOL Mg	SAFA Gm	FIBD Gm
Wine-cooler-white wine-7Up	serving	54.9	0.05	5.72	0	0	0	0
Water	cup	0	0	0	0	0	0	0
Lemon lime soda-7Up	fl oz	12.3	0	3.19	0	0	0	0
Tea-herb-brewed	fl oz	0.296	0	0.059	0	0	0.001	0
Gatorade-thirst quencher	fl oz	7.53	0	1.9	0	0	0	0
Tonic water-quinine soda	fl oz	10.4	0	2.68	0	0	0	0
Wine-rose-table	fl oz	20.9	0.059	0.413	0	0	0	0
BREADS								
Bagel-egg	item	163	6.02	30.9	1.41	8	-	1.16
Bagel-water	item	163	6.02	30.9	1.41	0	0.2	1.16
Biscuits-prepared/mix	item	104	1.63	13	5.05	1.4	3.31	0.504
Breadcrumbs-dry-grated	cup	390	13	73	5	0	1	3.65
Bread-cracked wheat	slice	65.5	2.32	12.5	0.868	0	0.1	1.33
Bread-french-enriched	slice	98	3.33	17.7	1.36	0	0.2	0.805
Bread-raisin-enriched	slice	69.5	2.05	13.2	0.99	0	0.2	0.55
Bread-rye-American-light	slice	65.5	2.12	12	0.913	0	-	1.55
Bread-pumpernickel	slice	81.6	2.93	15.4	1.1	0	-	1.89
Bread-white-firm	slice	61.4	1.9	11.2	0.902	0	0.2	0.437
Bread-white-firm-toasted	slice	65	2	12	1	0	0.2	0.5
Bread-whole wheat-firm	slice	61.3	2.41	11.3	1.09	0	0.1	2.83
Bread-wheat-firm toasted	slice	59	2.31	10.9	1.05	0	0.1	2.38
Crackers-Graham-plain	item	27.5	0.5	5	0.5	0	0.1	0.224
Crackers-rye wafers	item	22.5	1	5	0	0	0	1.05
Crackers-saltines	item	12.5	0.25	2	0.25	0.75	0.1	0.072

5

Food Name	Serving	KCAL Kc	PROT Gm	CARB Gm	FAT Gm	CHOL Mg	SAFA Gm	FIBD Gm
Muffin-blueberry-home rec	item	110	3	17	4	21	1.1	0.85
Muffin-bran-home rec	item	112	2.96	16.7	5.08	21	1.2	2.52
Muffin-corn-home rec	item	125	3	19	4	21	1.2	0.95
Muffin-plain-home rec	item	120	3	17	4	21	1	0.85
Pancakes-buckwheat-mix	item	55	2	6	2	20	0.8	0.621
Pancakes-plain-home recipe	item	60	2	9	2	20	0.5	0.45
Pancakes-plain-mix	item	58.9	1.85	7.87	2.17	20	0.7	0.394
Roll-brown & serve-enr	item	85	2	14	2	0	0.4	0.988
Roll-hamburger/hotdog	item	114	3.43	20.1	2.09	0	0.5	1.01
Roll-hard-enriched	item	155	5	30	2	0	0.4	1.5
Roll-submarine/hoagie-enr	item	390	12	75	4	0	0.9	3.75
Waffles-enr-home recipe	item	245	6.93	25.7	12.6	45	2.3	1.05
Muffin-English-plain	item	133	4.43	25.7	1.09	0	-	1.29
Muffin-English-plain-toast	item	154	5.13	29.8	1.26	0	-	1.49
Bread-corn-home rec	slice	108	2.21	15.6	3.94	0	-	1.17
Crackers-cheese	item	5.38	0.091	0.52	0.327	-	0.09	0.025
Crackers-graham-sug/honey	item	30.1	0.519	5.4	0.732	0	0.1	0.119
French toast-home recipe	slice	153	5.67	17.2	6.73	-	-	2.02
Waffles-frozen	item	103	2.15	15.9	3.52	0	-	0.888
Bread-mixed grain	slice	64.3	2.49	11.7	0.93	0	-	1.58
Bread-whole wheat-home rec	slice	66.5	2.25	11.6	1.61	0	-	2.83
Bread-pita	item	105	3.95	20.6	0.57	0	-	0.608
Crackers-Flykrisp-natural	item	7.5	0.25	1.67	0.033	0	0	0.34
Crackers-animal	item	8.67	0.127	1.47	0.2	0	-	0.027
Crackers-cheddar snacks	item	7.22	0.144	1.11	0.261	-	-	0.056
Crackers-triscuits	item	21	0.4	3.1	0.75	0	-	0.155

Food Name	Serving	KCAL Kc	PROT Gm	CARB Gm	FAT Gm	CHOL Mg	SAFA Gm	FIBD Gm
Crackers-wheat thins	item	9	0.125	1.25	0.35	0	-	0.099
Roll-whole wheat-homemade	item	90	3.5	18.3	1	0	-	1.83
Croissant-roll-Sara Lee	item	109	2.3	11.2	6.1	-	-	0.56
Muffin-soy	item	119	3.9	16.7	4.4	0	-	0.835
Bread stick-vienna type	item	106	3.3	20.3	1.1	0	-	1.02
Crackers-Ritz	item	18	0.233	2.13	0.967	0	-	0.107
BREAKFAST CEREALS								
Cereal-corn grits-enriched	cup	145	3.39	31.5	0.484	0	0.073	0.6
Cereal-farina-cook-enr	cup	117	3.26	24.7	0.233	0	0.023	3.26
Cereal-wheat-rolled-cooked	cup	180	5	41	1	0	0.182	2.87
Cereal-wheat-whole meal	cup	110	4	23	1	0	0.182	1.61
Cereal-frost flake-Kellogg	cup	133	1.75	31.7	0.07	0	0	0.77
Cereal-corn-shredded sugar	cup	95	2	22	0	0	0	1.54
Cereal-oats-puffed-sugar	cup	100	3	19	1	0	0.185	2.65
Cereal-rice-puffed-plain	cup	56.3	0.882	12.6	0.07	0	0	0.1
Cereal-rice-puffed-sugar	cup	115	1	26	0	0	0	0.2
Cereal-wheat flakes-sugar	cup	105	3	24	0	0	0	2.7
Cereal-wheat-puffed plain	cup	43.7	1.76	9.55	0.144	0	-	0.4
Cereal-wheat-puffed-sugar	serving	138	5.59	30.2	0.456	0	0	2.11
Cereal-wheat-shred-biscuit	item	83	2.6	18.8	0.3	0	0	2.2
Cereal-wheat germ-toasted	cup	432	32.9	56.1	12.1	0	2.07	14.6
Cereal-cream/wheat-packet	item	132	2.5	28.9	0.4	0	0	2.02
Cereal-oatmeal-inst packet	item	104	4.4	18.1	1.7	0	0.289	1.62
Cereal-Ralston-cooked	cup	134	5.57	28.2	0.8	0	0	4.2
Cereal-All Bran	cup	212	12.2	63.4	1.53	0	-	25.5

Food Name	Serving	KCAL Kc	PROT Gm	CARB Gm	FAT Gm	CHOL Mg	SAFA Gm	FIBD Gm
Cereal-Alpha Bits	cup	111	2.2	24.6	0.6	0	-	0.3
Cereal-Bran Buds	cup	220	11.8	64.8	2.04	0	-	23.6
Cereal-Bran Chex	cup	156	5.05	39	1.37	0	-	7.9
Cereal-C.W. Post-plain	cup	432	8.7	69.4	15.2	0.184	11.3	2.2
Cereal-Cheerios	cup	88.8	3.42	15.7	1.45	0	0.27	0.863
Cereal-corn bran	cup	125	2.45	30.3	1.26	0	-	6.84
Cereal-Corn Chex	cup	111	2.02	24.9	0.114	0	0	0.5
Cereal-corn flakes-Kellogg	cup	88.3	1.84	19.5	0.068	0	0	0.454
Cereal-Cracklin Bran	cup	229	5.52	41.2	8.76	0	-	9.1
Cereal-Crispy rice	cup	112	1.82	25.2	0.114	0	0	1
Cereal-fortified oat flake	cup	177	8.98	34.8	0.72	0	0	1.2
Cereal-bran flakes-Kellogg	cup	127	4.91	30.5	0.741	0	0	5.5
Cereal-Frosted Mini Wheats	item	25.5	0.731	5.86	0.071	0	0	0.54
Cereal-Granola-homemade	cup	594	15	67.3	33.2	0	5.84	12.8
Cereal-Grape Nuts	cup	407	13.3	93.5	0.456	0	0	5.47
Cereal-Grape Nuts Flakes	cup	116	3.48	26.6	0.358	0	0	2.08
Cereal-Heartland Natural	cup	499	11.6	78.5	17.7	0	-	5.4
Cereal-Honey Nut Cheerios	cup	125	3.63	26.5	0.759	0	0.132	1.3
Cereal-Honey Bran	cup	119	3.08	28.6	0.735	0	0	3.9
Cereal-Life-plain/cinnamon	cup	162	8.1	31.5	0.836	0	0	1.4
Cereal-Lucky Charms	cup	125	2.91	26.1	1.22	0	0.224	0.6
Cereal-granola-Nature Val	cup	503	11.5	75.5	19.6	0	13	4.2
Cereal-Nutri Grain-barley	cup	153	4.47	33.9	0.328	0	0	2.4
Cereal-Nutri Grain-corn	cup	160	3.36	35.4	0.966	0	-	2.6
Cereal-Nutri Grain-rye	cup	144	3.48	33.9	0.28	0	0	2.56
Cereal-Nutri Grain-wheat	cup	158	3.83	37.2	0.44	0	0	2.8

Food Name	Serving	KCAL Kc	PROT Gm	CARB Gm	FAT Gm	CHOL Mg	SAFA Gm	FIBD Gm
Cereal-100% bran	cup	178	8.25	48.1	3.3	0	0.587	19.5
Cereal-Product 19	cup	126	3.23	27.4	0.231	0	0	0.4
Cereal-Raisin Bran-Kellogg	cup	154	5.31	37.1	0.984	0	-	5.31
Cereal-Rice Chex	cup	99.5	1.34	22.5	0.101	0	0	0.151
Cereal-Rice Krispies	cup	112	1.93	24.8	0.199	0	0	0.1
Cereal-Special K	cup	83.1	4.2	16	0.085	0.028	0	0.17
Cereal-Sugar Corn Pops	cup	108	1.42	25.7	0.085	0	0	0.2
Cereal-Sugar Smacks	cup	141	2.65	33	0.72	0	0	0.531
Cereal-Team	cup	164	2.69	36	0.756	0	0	0.7
Cereal-Toasties	cup	87.8	1.84	19.5	0.045	0	0	0.386
Cereal-Total	cup	116	3.3	26	0.693	0	0.099	2.4
Cereal-Trix	cup	109	1.53	25.2	0.398	0	0	0.32
Cereal-Wheat Chex	cup	169	4.55	37.8	1.15	0	-	3.4
Cereal-wheat germ-sugar	cup	426	24.6	68.7	9.04	0	1.57	5.7
Cereal-Wheaties	cup	101	2.8	23.1	0.5	0	0.07	2
Cereal-cream/wheat-reg-hot	cup	133	3.8	27.7	0.5	0	0	1.94
Cereal-cream/wheat-instant	cup	153	4.4	31.6	0.6	0	0	2.21
Cereal-malt o meal-cook	cup	122	3.6	25.9	0.24	0	0	0.6
Cereal-Maypo-cook-hot	cup	170	5.8	31.8	2.4	0	-	1.2
Cereal-Roman Meal-cooked	cup	147	6.51	33	0.964	0	0	2.31
Cereal-Wheatena-cooked	cup	136	4.86	28.7	1.22	0	-	2.6
Cereal-whole wheat natural	cup	150	4.84	33.2	0.968	0	-	2.7
Cereal-oatmeal-raw	cup	311	13	54.2	5.1	0	0.9	4.6

Food Name	Serving	KCAL Kc	PROT Gm	CARB Gm	FAT Gm	CHOL Mg	SAFA Gm	FIBD Gm
COMBINATION FOODS								
Beef-raviolios-canned	ounce	27.5	1.14	4.26	0.568	-	0.11	0.23
Salad-three-bean-Del Monte	ounce	22.4	0.71	5.06	0.056	0	0	1.52
Salad-tuna	cup	350	30	7	22	68	4.3	1.03
Beef-vegetable stew	cup	220	16	15	11	72	4.9	3.19
Beef potpie-home recipe	slice	515	21	39	30	44	7.9	3.9
Chili concarne /beans-can	cup	340	19	31	16	38	7.5	5
Chicken a la king-home rec	cup	470	27	12	34	186	12.9	1.2
Chicken chow mein-canned	cup	95	7	18	0	98	0	0.9
Chicken potpie-baked-home	slice	545	23	42	31	72	11	4.2
Macaroni & cheese-enr-can	cup	230	9	26	10	42	4.2	1.44
Macaroni & cheese-enr-home	cup	430	17	40	22	42	8.9	1.2
Pizza-cheese-baked	slice	140	7.68	20.5	3.21	9	1.54	1.59
Spaghetti/tom/che-home rec	cup	260	9	37	9	4	2	2.5
Spaghetti/tom/che-can	cup	190	6	39	2	4	0.5	2.5
Spaghetti/tom/meat-home	cup	330	19	39	12	75	3.3	2.73
Spaghetti/tom/meat-can	cup	260	12	29	10	39	2.2	2.75
Beans/pork/frankfurter-can	cup	365	17.3	39.6	16.9	15.4	6.05	12.8
Beans/pork/tom sauce-can	cup	248	13.1	49.1	2.61	17	0.999	13.8
Beans/pork/sweet sauce-can	cup	281	13.4	53.1	3.69	17.7	1.42	14
Salad-potato	cup	358	6.7	27.9	20.5	170	3.57	5.25
Vegetables-mixed-froz-boil	cup	107	5.21	23.8	0.273	0	0.056	6.92
Salad-fruit-can/juice	cup	125	1.27	32.5	0.075	0	0.01	1.64
Salad-coleslaw	tbsp	5.52	0.103	0.993	0.209	1	0.031	0.297
Taco	item	370	20.7	26.7	20.6	57	11.4	2.67

Food Name	Serving	KCAL Kc	PROT Gm	CARB Gm	FAT Gm	CHOL Mg	SAFA Gm	FIBD Gm
Pizza-pepperoni-baked	slice	181	10.1	19.9	6.96	14	2.24	1.48
Sand-bac/let/tom/mayo	item	282	6.8	28.8	15.6	-	-	2.88
Sandwich-club	item	590	35.6	41.7	20.8	-	-	4.17
Salad-macaroni	serving	50.7	0.7	5.3	5.3	-	-	0.29
Salad-carrot raisin-home	cup	306	3.8	55.8	11.6	-	-	16.7
Salad-mandarin orange gel	serving	22.7	0.4	5.7	0	0	0	0.57
Salad-chicken	cup	502	26	17.4	36.2	-	-	-
Chili with beans-canned	cup	286	14.6	30.4	14	43.4	6	6.93
Salad-green salad-tossed	serving	32	2.6	6.67	0.16	0	0.021	2.11
Meat loaf-celery/onions	serving	213	15.8	5.23	13.9	107	5.29	0.11
Salad-chef salad-ham/chees	serving	196	13.4	7.42	12.7	46	6.98	2.39
DAIRY PRODUCTS								
Cheese-blue	ounce	100	6.06	0.659	8.14	21	5.29	0
Cheese-camembert-wedge	item	114	7.52	0.18	9.22	27	5.8	0
Cheese-cheddar-shredded	cup	455	28.1	1.45	37.5	119	23.8	0
Cheese-cottage-4% lar curd	cup	232	28.1	6.03	10.1	33.8	6.41	0
Cheese-cream	ounce	100	2.17	0.759	10	31.4	6.31	0
Cheese-mozzarella-skim milk	ounce	72	6.88	0.78	4.51	16	2.87	0
Cheese-parmesan-grated	cup	456	41.6	3.74	30	79	19.1	0
Cheese-provolone	ounce	100	7.25	0.61	7.55	20	4.84	0
Cheese-ricotta-skim milk	cup	340	28	12.6	19.5	76	12.1	0
Cheese-romano	ounce	110	9.02	1.03	7.64	29	4.85	0
Cheese-Swiss	ounce	107	8.06	0.96	7.78	26	5.04	0
Cheese-American-processed	ounce	106	6.28	0.45	8.86	27	5.58	0

11

Food Name	Serving	KCAL Kc	PROT Gm	CARB Gm	FAT Gm	CHOL Mg	SAFA Gm	FIBD Gm
Cheese-Swiss-processed	ounce	95	7.01	0.6	7.09	24	4.55	0
Cheese food-American-proc	ounce	93	5.56	2.07	6.97	18	4.38	0
Cheese-spread-processed	ounce	82	4.65	2.48	6.02	16	3.78	0
Cream-half & half-fluid	cup	315	7.16	10.4	27.8	89	17.3	0
Cream-coffee-table -light	cup	469	6.48	8.78	46.3	159	28.9	0
Cream-whipping-heavy	cup	821	4.88	6.64	88.1	326	54.8	0
Cream-whip-pressurized	cup	154	1.92	7.49	13.3	46	8.3	0
Cream-sour-cultured	cup	493	7.27	9.82	48.2	102	30	0
Cream-whip-imit-froz	cup	239	0.94	17.3	19	0	16.3	0
Cream-whip-imit-pressurize	cup	184	0.69	11.3	15.6	0	13.2	0
Milk-whole-3.3% fat-fluid	cup	150	8.03	11.4	8.15	33	5.07	0
Milk-2% fat-lowfat-fluid	cup	121	8.12	11.7	4.68	18	2.92	0
Milk-2% milk solids added	cup	125	8.53	12.2	4.7	18	2.93	0
Milk 1% fat-lowfat-fluid	cup	102	8.03	11.7	2.59	10	1.61	0
Milk-buttermilk-fluid	cup	99	8.11	11.7	2.16	9	1.34	0
Milk-evaporated-whole can	cup	338	17.2	25.3	19.1	73.1	11.6	0
Milk-evaporated-skim can	cup	199	19.3	28.9	0.51	10.2	0.309	0
Milk-condensed-sweet can	cup	982	24.2	166	26.6	104	16.8	0
Milk-chocolate-whole	cup	208	7.92	25.9	8.48	30	5.26	0.15
Milk-eggnog-commercial	cup	342	9.68	34.4	19	149	11.3	0
Milkshake-chocolate-thick	item	356	9.15	63.5	8.1	32	5.04	0.75
Milkshake-vanilla-thick	item	350	12.1	55.6	9.48	37	5.9	0.2
Yogurt-fruit flavor-lowfat	cup	231	9.92	43.2	2.45	10	1.58	0.2
Yogurt-plain-lowfat	cup	144	11.9	16	3.52	14	2.27	0.8
Yogurt-plain-nonfat	cup	127	13	17.4	0.41	4	0.264	0
Yogurt-plain-whole	cup	139	7.88	10.6	7.38	29	4.76	0

Food Name	Serving	KCAL Kc	PROT Gm	CARB Gm	FAT Gm	CHOL Mg	SAFA Gm	FIBD Gm
Cheese-feta	ounce	75	4.03	1.16	6.03	25	4.24	0
Cheese-gouda	ounce	101	7.07	0.63	7.78	32	4.99	0
Cheese-limburger	ounce	93	5.68	0.14	7.72	26	4.75	0
Cheese-monterey	ounce	106	6.94	0.19	8.58	25.2	5.41	0
Cheese-roquefort	ounce	105	6.11	0.57	8.69	26	5.46	0
Cream-sour-half & half	tbsp	20	0.44	0.64	1.8	6	1.12	0
Cream-sour-imitation	ounce	59	0.68	1.88	5.53	0	5.04	0
Milk-whole-low sodium	cup	149	7.56	10.9	8.44	33	5.26	0
Milk-human-whole-mature	cup	171	2.53	17	10.8	34	4.94	0
DESSERTS								
Ice cream-van-hard-10% fat	cup	269	4.8	31.7	14.3	59	8.92	0
Ice cream-van-soft serve	cup	377	7.04	38.3	22.5	153	13.5	0
Ice milk-van-soft-2.6% fat	cup	223	8.03	38.4	4.62	13	2.88	0
Sherbet-orange-2% fat	cup	270	2.16	58.7	3.82	14	2.38	0
Custard-baked	cup	305	14	29	15	278	6.8	1.02
Pudd-tapioca cream-home	cup	220	8	28	8	80	4.1	0.56
Pudd-choc-cooked-mix/milk	cup	320	9	59	8	32	4.3	0
Pudd-choc-inst-mix/milk	cup	325	8	63	7	28	3.6	0
Cake-angelfood-mix/prep	slice	142	4.2	31.5	0.122	0	-	0.037
Cupcake/chocolate icing	item	130	2	21	5	15	2	0.42
Cake-gingerbread-mix/prep	slice	175	2	32	4	1	1.1	1.83
Cake-yellow/icing-home rec	slice	268	2.9	40.3	11.4	36	3	0.552
Cake-fruit-dark-home rec	slice	56.9	0.72	8.96	2.3	6.75	0.48	0.313
Cake-sheet-no icing-home	slice	315	4	48	12	1	3.3	0.96

13

Food Name	Serving	KCAL Kc	PROT Gm	CARB Gm	FAT Gm	CHOL Mg	SAFA Gm	FIBD Gm
Cake-pound-home recipe	slice	160	2	16	10	68	54.9	0.08
Cake-sponge-home recipe	slice	188	4.82	35.7	3.14	162	1.1	0
Cookie-chocolate chip-mix	item	50	0.5	6.96	2.42	5.52	0.7	0.284
Cookie-choc chip-home rec	item	46.3	0.5	6.41	2.68	5.25	0.6	0.27
Cookie-macaroon	item	90	1	12.5	4.5	0	-	0.437
Cookie-oatmeal/raisin-mix	item	61.5	0.732	8.93	2.6	0	0.5	0.351
Cookie-sandwich-choc/van	item	50	0.5	7	2.25	0	0.55	0.15
Cookie-vanilla wafer	item	18.5	0.2	3	0.6	2.5	0.1	0.01
Danish pastry-plain	item	250	4.06	29.1	13.6	0	4.7	0.582
Doughnuts-cake-plain	item	104	1.28	12.2	5.77	10	1.2	0.325
Doughnuts-yeast-glazed	item	205	3	22	11.2	13	3	1.1
Pie-apple-home rec	slice	323	2.75	49.1	13.6	0	3.9	2.16
Pie-banana cream-home rec	slice	285	6	40	12	40	3.8	1.4
Pie-cherry-home rec	slice	350	4	52	15	0	4	1.08
Pie-custard-home rec	slice	285	8	30	14	-	4.8	2.08
Pie-lemon meringue-home rec	slice	300	3.86	47.3	11.2	0	3.7	1.44
Pie-mince-home rec	slice	365	3	56	16	0	4	1.96
Pie-peach-home rec	slice	345	3	52	14	0	3.5	1.82
Pie-pecan-home rec	slice	495	6	61	27	0	4	4.13
Pie-pumpkin-home rec	slice	275	5	32	15	0	5.4	3.51
Piecrust-mix/prep-baked	item	743	10	70.5	46.5	0	11.4	4.23
Granola bar	item	109	2.35	16	4.23	-	0.96	0.96
Cookie-sugar-mix	item	98.8	0.908	13.1	4.79	-	-	0.262
Cake-cheesecake-commercial	slice	257	4.61	24.3	16.3	-	-	1.79
Ice cream sundae-hot fudge	item	297	5.89	49.8	9.01	21.5	5.25	-
Turnover-apple	ounce	85.2	0.738	10.5	4.71	1.42	-	0.21

Food Name	Serving	KCAL Kc	PROT Gm	CARB Gm	FAT Gm	CHOL Mg	SAFA Gm	FIBD Gm
Cookie-peanut butter-mix	item	50	0.8	5.87	2.64	-	-	0.18
Pudd-rice/raisins	cup	387	9.5	70.8	8.2	-	-	1.42
Cake-strawberry shortcake	serving	344	4.8	61.2	8.9	-	-	2.14
Froz yogurt-fruit variety cup		216	7	41.8	2	-	-	-
Twinkie-Hostess	item	143	1.25	25.6	4.2	21	-	-
EGGS								
Egg-whole-raw-large	item	75	6.25	0.61	5.01	213	1.55	0
Egg-white-raw-large	item	17	3.52	0.34	0	0	0	0
Egg-yolk-raw-large	item	59	2.78	0.3	5.12	213	1.59	0
Egg-hard-large-no shell	item	77	6.29	0.56	5.3	213	1.63	0
Egg-poached-large-large	item	74	6.22	0.61	4.99	212	1.54	0
Egg-substitute-liquid	cup	211	30.1	1.61	8.31	2.51	1.65	0
FATS/OILS								
Butter-regular-tablespoon	tbsp	100	0.119	0.008	11.4	30.7	7.07	0
Butter-whipped-tablespoon	tbsp	64.5	0.077	0.005	7.3	19.7	4.54	0
Shortening-vegetable-soy	cup	1812	0	0	205	0	51.2	0
Margarine-diet mazola	tbsp	50	0	0	5.7	0	1	0
Margarine-veg spray-Mazola	serving	6	0	0	0.72	0	0.08	0
Margarine-reg-hard-stick	item	812	1.02	1.02	91	0	17.9	0
Vegetable oil-corn	cup	1927	0	0	218	0	27.7	0
Vegetable oil-olive	cup	1909	0	0	216	0	29.2	0
Sal dress-blue cheese	tbsp	77.1	0.7	1.1	8	2.6	1.5	0.05

Food Name	Serving	KCAL Kc	PROT Gm	CARB Gm	FAT Gm	CHOL Mg	SAFA Gm	FIBD Gm
Sal dress-blue che-low cal	tbsp	10	0	1	1	4	0.5	0
Sal dress-French	tbsp	67	0.1	2.7	6.4	1.95	1.5	0.1
Sal Dress-French-low cal	tbsp	21.9	0.033	3.5	0.9	0.978	0.13	0.09
Sal dress-Italian	tbsp	68.7	0	1.5	7.1	0	1	0.05
Sal dress-Italian-low cal	tbsp	15.8	0	0.7	1.5	1	0.2	0.09
Sal dress-mayonnaise type	tbsp	57.3	0.132	4.91	4.91	3.82	0.72	0
Sal Dress-mayo-low cal	tbsp	20	0	2	2	2	0.4	0
Sal dress-thousand Island	tbsp	58.9	0.14	2.4	5.6	4.9	0.9	0.6
Sal dress-thous isl-low cal	tbsp	24.3	0.1	2.5	1.6	2	0.2	0.3
Animal fat-cooking-chicken	tbsp	115	0	0	12.8	11	3.8	0
Margarine-corn-reg-hard	tsp	33.8	0	0	3.8	0	0.6	0
Margarine-corn-reg-soft	tsp	33.7	0	0	3.8	0	0.7	0
Mayonnaise-imitation-soy	tbsp	34.7	0.045	2.4	2.9	3.6	0.495	0
Sal dress-Russian-low cal	tbsp	23	0.082	4.5	0.652	1	0.1	0.2
Sal dress-Russian	tbsp	76	0.2	1.6	7.8	0	1.1	0
Sal dress-vinegar/oil-home	tbsp	70	0	0.39	7.81	0	1.42	0
Sandwich spread-commercial	tbsp	59.5	0.1	3.4	5.2	12	0.8	0.02
Mayonnaise-light-low cal	tbsp	40	0	1	4	5	-	0
Miracle whip-light-low cal	tbsp	45	0	2	4	5	-	0
Sal dress-caesar	tbsp	70	0	1	7	-	-	0.04
Sal dress-ranch style	tbsp	54	0.4	0.6	5.7	-	-	0
FISH								
Fish-bluefish-baked/butter	item	246	40.6	0	8.1	108	1.83	0
Fish-clams-raw-meat only	serving	62.9	10.9	2.18	0.83	28.9	0.08	0

Food Name	Serving	KCAL Kc	PROT Gm	CARB Gm	FAT Gm	CHOL Mg	SAFA Gm	FIBD Gm
Fish-clam-can-solid/liquid	ounce	12.8	2.33	0.667	0.333	17.7	0.067	0
Fish-crab meat-king-can	cup	135	24	1	3.2	135	0.6	0
Fish-stick-bread-froz-cook	ounce	77.2	4.44	6.75	3.47	31.8	0.894	0.665
Fish-perch-breaded-fried	piece	195	16	6	11	32	2.7	0.05
Fish-oysters-raw-meat only	cup	171	17.5	9.7	6.14	136	1.56	0
Fish-salmon-pink-can	serving	118	16.8	0	5.14	46.8	1.3	0
Fish-sardines-can/oil	item	25	2.95	0	1.37	17	0.184	0
Fish-shad-bake/marg/bacon	serving	201	23.2	0	11.3	69.4	2.45	0
Fish-shrimp-meat-can	cup	154	29.5	1.32	2.51	221	0.477	0
Fish-shrimp-french fried	serving	206	18.2	9.75	10.4	150	1.77	0.48
Fish-tuna-can/oil-drained	serving	168	24.8	0	6.98	15.3	1.3	0
Fish-tuna-white can/water	serving	116	22.7	0	2.09	35.7	0.556	0
Fish-tuna-diet-low sodium	ounce	35.5	7.67	0.011	0.54	9.94	0.09	0
Fish-tuna-light-can/water	serving	111	25.1	0	0.525	15.3	0.136	0
Fish-anchovy-fillet can	item	8.4	1.16	0	0.388	3.4	0.088	0
Fish-cod-cooked-dry heat	piece	189	41.1	0	1.55	99	0.302	0
Fish-crab cake	item	93	12.1	0.288	4.51	90	0.89	0.03
Fish-crab-steamed pieces	cup	150	30	0	2.39	82.2	0.206	0
Fish-sole-/flounder-baked	serving	148	30.7	0	1.94	86	0.461	0
Fish-haddock-cook-dry heat	serving	95.2	20.6	0	0.79	62.9	0.142	0
Fish-mackerel-Atlantic-can	cup	296	44.1	0	12	150	3.53	0
Fish-rockfish-ckd-dry heat	serving	121	24	0	2.01	44	0.474	0
Fish-roe-raw-eggs	ounce	39.4	6.34	0.426	1.82	106	0.414	0
Fish-salmon-smoked	serving	117	18.3	0	4.32	23	0.929	0
Fish-scallops-steamed	ounce	31.8	6.59	0.511	0.398	15.1	-	0
Fish-swordfish-broil/marg	serving	174	28	0	6	4	-	0

Food Name	Serving	KCAL Kc	PROT Gm	CARB Gm	FAT Gm	CHOL Mg	SAFA Gm	FIBD Gm
Fish-trout-brook-cooked	serving	196	23.5	0.4	11.2	-	-	0
Fish-whitefish-bake/stuff	serving	215	15.2	5.8	14	-	-	0.58
Fish-white perch-fri-filet	item	108	12.5	0	5.3	-	-	0
Fish-carp-cooked-dry heat	serving	138	19.4	0	6.1	71.4	1.18	0
Fish-catfish-fried-breaded	serving	195	15.4	6.83	11.3	68.9	2.79	0.8
Fish-flatfish-ckd-dry heat	serving	99.5	20.5	0	1.3	58	0.309	0
Fish-grouper-ckd-dry heat	serving	100	25.7	0	1.11	40	0.254	0
Fish-mackerel-ckd-dry heat	serving	223	20.3	0	15.1	63.8	3.55	0
Fish-ocean perch-ckd-dry	serving	103	20.3	0	1.78	45.9	0.266	0
Fish-perch-cooked-dry heat	serving	99.5	21.1	0	1	98	0.201	0
Fish-pollock-ckd-dry heat	serving	96.1	20	0	0.952	81.6	0.196	0
Fish-pompano-ckd-dry heat	serving	179	20.1	0	10.3	54.4	3.82	0
Fish-salmon-ckd-moist heat	serving	157	23.3	0	6.41	41.7	1.19	0
Fish-sea-bass-ckd-dry heat	serving	105	20.1	0	2.18	45.1	0.557	0
Fish-smelt-cooked-dry heat	serving	105	19.2	0	2.64	76.5	0.492	0
Fish-red snapper-ckd-dry	serving	109	22.4	0	1.46	40	0.31	0
Fish-surimi	serving	84.2	12.9	5.82	0.765	25.5	0.153	0
Fish-pollock-atlantic-raw	serving	78.2	16.5	0	0.833	60.4	0.115	0
Fish-swordfish-cooked-dry	serving	132	21.6	0	4.37	42.5	1.2	0
Fish-trout-rainbow-ckd-dry	serving	128	22.4	0	3.66	62.1	0.707	0
Fish-tuna-yellowfin-raw	serving	91.8	19.9	0	0.81	38.3	0.2	0
Fish-whiting-ckd-dry heat	serving	98	20	0	1.43	71.4	0.269	0
Fish-crab-imitation-surimi	serving	86.7	10.2	8.69	1.11	17	0.221	0
Fish-crayfish-ckd-moist	serving	96.9	20.3	0	1.15	151	0.197	0
Fish-lobster-ckd-moist	ounce	27.8	5.82	0.364	0.168	20.4	0.03	0
Fish-shrimp-ckd-moist heat	serving	84.2	17.8	0	0.918	166	0.246	0

Food Name	Serving	KCAL Kc	PROT Gm	CARB Gm	FAT Gm	CHOL Mg	SAFA Gm	FIBD Gm
Fish-clams-breaded-fried	serving	172	12.1	8.78	8.78	51.9	2.28	0.32
Fish-clams-ckd-moist heat	serving	126	21.7	4.36	1.65	57	0.16	0
Fish-mussel-blue-ckd-moist	serving	147	20.2	6.28	3.81	47.6	0.723	0
Fish-oyster-Eastern-canned	cup	171	17.5	9.7	6.14	136	1.57	0
Fish-oyster-east-ckd-moist	serving	117	12	6.65	4.21	92.7	1.07	0
Fish-oysters-pacific-raw	serving	68.9	8.03	4.21	1.96	42.5	0.434	0
Fish-squid-cooked-fried	serving	149	15.3	6.62	6.36	221	1.6	0.3
Fish-halibut-broiled-dry	serving	119	22.7	0	2.5	34.9	0.354	0

FROZEN DINNERS

Food Name	Serving	KCAL Kc	PROT Gm	CARB Gm	FAT Gm	CHOL Mg	SAFA Gm	FIBD Gm
Fish divan-Lean Cuisine	item	270	31	16	10	85	-	-
Fettucini alfredo-Stouffer	item	270	8	19	18	-	-	-
Turkey pie-Stouffer	item	460	20	35	26	-	-	-
Meatballs/noodles-Stouffer	item	475	25	33	27	-	-	-
Beef/green peppers-Stouf	item	225	10	18	11	-	-	-
Lasagna-Stouffer	item	385	28	36	14	-	-	-
Chicken cacciatore-Stouf	item	310	25	29	11	-	-	-
Veal parmigiana-froz din	item	296	24	17	14	-	-	-
Cabbage roll/tom sauc-horm	ounce	23	1.1	3.2	0.7	3	0.281	-
Chicken kiev-Le Menu	item	500	21	35	30	-	-	-
Vegetable lasagna- Le Menu	item	400	15	30	24	-	-	-
Beef sirloin tips-Le Menu	item	400	29	27	19	-	-	-
Chicken parmigiana-Le Menu	item	390	26	28	19	-	-	-
Manicotti-cheese-Le Menu	item	310	18	29	13	-	-	-
Sole-light-Van de Kamps	item	293	16	17	18	-	-	-

19

Food Name	Serving	KCAL Kc	PROT Gm	CARB Gm	FAT Gm	CHOL Mg	SAFA Gm	FIBD Gm
Mexican dinner-Swanson	item	590	20	64	29	-	-	-
Beef dinner-Swanson	item	320	25	34	9	-	-	-
Turkey dinner-Swanson	item	340	20	42	10	-	-	-
Chicken dinner-Swanson	item	660	26	64	33	-	-	-
Egg roll-beef/shrimp/froz	item	27	0.9	3.5	1	-	-	0.12
Fish & chips-Van de Kamps	item	500	16	45	30	-	-	-
Meatloaf-froz din-Banquet	item	412	20.9	29	23.7	-	-	-
Ham-froz din-Banquet	item	369	16.8	47.7	12.2	-	-	-
Salisbury steak din-Banq	item	390	18.1	24	24.6	-	-	-
FRUITS								
Apples-raw-unpeeled	item	81	0.262	21.1	0.497	0	0.08	3.04
Apple juice-canned/bottled	cup	116	0.15	29	0.28	0	0.047	0.52
Applesauce-can-sweetened	cup	194	0.459	50.8	0.47	0	0.077	3.06
Applesauce-can-unsweetened	cup	105	0.415	27.6	0.12	0	0.02	3.66
Apricot-raw-without pit	item	16.9	0.494	3.93	0.138	0	0.01	0.67
Apricots-dried-uncooked	cup	309	4.75	80.3	0.6	0	0.042	10.1
Apricots-dried-cooked-unsw	cup	213	3.24	54.8	0.4	0	0.028	19.5
Avocado-raw-California	item	306	3.65	12	30	0	4.48	6.13
Bananas-raw-peeled	item	105	1.17	26.7	0.547	0	0.211	1.82
Blackberries-raw	cup	74.9	1.04	18.4	0.562	0	0.07	8.93
Blueberries-raw	cup	81.2	0.972	20.5	0.551	0	0.07	3.34
Cherries-sweet-raw	item	4.9	0.082	1.13	0.065	0	0.015	0.1
Cranberry sauce-can-sweet	cup	418	0.554	108	0.416	0	0.06	3.2
Dates-natural-dried-chop	cup	490	3.51	131	0.801	0	0.05	15.5

20

Food Name	Serving	KCAL Kc	PROT Gm	CARB Gm	FAT Gm	CHOL Mg	SAFA Gm	FBD Gm
Grapefruit-raw-pink & red	item	74	1.36	18.5	0.246	0	0.034	3.2
Grapefruit-raw-white	item	78	1.63	19.8	0.236	0	0.033	2.5
Grapefruit juice-raw	cup	96.3	1.24	22.7	0.247	0	0.035	0.5
Grapefruit juice-can-uns	cup	93.9	1.28	22.1	0.247	0	0.032	0.442
Grapefruit juice-can-sweet	cup	115	1.45	27.8	0.225	0	0.03	0
Grapefruit juice-froz-dilu	cup	101	1.36	24	0.321	0	0.047	0
Grape juice-can & bottle	cup	154	1.42	37.8	0.202	0	0.063	0
Grape juice-froz-diluted	cup	128	0.475	31.9	0.225	0	0.073	0
Grape drink-canned	cup	154	1.42	37.8	0.202	0	0.063	0
Lemons-raw-peeled	item	16.8	0.638	5.41	0.174	0	0.023	0.58
Lemon juice-raw	cup	61	0.927	21.1	0	0	0	0.732
Lemon juice-can & bottle	cup	51.2	0.976	15.8	0.708	0	0.093	0.732
Lemonade-froz-diluted	cup	105	0	28	0	0	0	0.56
lime juice-raw	cup	66.4	1.08	22.2	0.246	0	0.027	0
Lime juice-can & bottle	cup	51.7	0.615	16.5	0.566	0	0.064	0
Melons-cantaloupe-raw	cup	56	1.41	13.4	0.448	0	0	1.28
Melons-honeydew-raw	cup	59.5	0.782	15.6	0.17	0	0.02	1.53
Oranges-raw-all varieties	item	61.6	1.23	15.4	0.157	0	0.02	3.14
Orange juice-raw	cup	111	1.74	25.8	0.496	0	0.06	1.98
Orange juice-can	cup	104	1.47	24.5	0.349	0	0.045	0.26
Orange juice-froz-diluted	cup	112	1.69	26.8	0.149	0	0.017	0.498
Papayas-raw	cup	54.6	0.854	13.7	0.196	0	0.06	1.27
Peaches-raw-whole	item	37.4	0.609	9.66	0.078	0	0.009	1.39
Peaches-raw-sliced	cup	73.1	1.19	18.9	0.153	0	0.017	2.72
Peaches-can/water pack	cup	58.6	1.07	14.9	0.146	0	0.015	1.08
Peaches-dried-uncooked	cup	382	5.78	98.1	1.22	0	0.131	14

Food Name	Serving	KCAL Kc	PROT Gm	CARB Gm	FAT Gm	CHOL Mg	SAFA Gm	FIBD Gm
Peaches-dried-cooked-uns	cup	199	2.99	50.8	0.645	0	0.067	6.7
Peaches-froz-sliced-sweet	cup	235	1.58	60	0.33	0	0.035	5.99
Pears-raw-bartlett-unpeeled	item	97.9	0.647	25.1	0.664	0	0.037	4.32
Pineapple-raw-diced	cup	76	0.605	19.2	0.667	0	0.05	1.86
Pineapple juice-can	cup	140	0.8	34.5	0.2	0	0.013	0.25
Plums-raw-prune type	item	20	0	6	0	0	0	0.588
Prunes-dried-uncooked	cup	385	4.2	101	0.837	0	0.066	11
Prune juice-can & bottle	cup	182	1.56	44.7	0.077	0	0.008	2.56
Raisins-seedless	cup	435	4.67	115	0.667	0	0.218	7.69
Raisins-seedless-packet	item	42	0.451	11.1	0.064	0	0.021	0.742
Raspberries-raw	cup	60.3	1.12	14.2	0.677	0	0.023	5.5
Rhubarb-raw-cooked-sugar	cup	380	1	97	0	0	0	5.4
Strawberries-raw-whole	cup	44.7	0.909	10.5	0.551	0	0.03	3.87
Tangerines-raw-peeled	item	37	0.53	9.4	0.16	0	0.018	1.68
Watermelon-raw	cup	51.2	0.992	11.5	0.688	0	-	0.64
Apples-raw-peeled-boiled	cup	90.6	0.45	23.3	0.61	0	0.099	4.1
Apple juice-frozen-diluted	cup	112	0.34	27.6	0.239	0	0.043	0.55
Apricots-can/juice	cup	119	1.56	30.6	0.09	0	0.007	2.81
Blackberries-frozen-unsw	cup	96.6	1.78	23.7	0.649	0	-	7.55
Blueberries-frozen-unsweet	cup	79.1	0.651	18.9	0.992	0	-	4.94
Boysenberries-frozen-unsw	cup	66	1.45	16.1	0.343	0	-	5.15
Figs-dried-uncooked	cup	507	6.07	130	2.33	0	0.466	18.5
Fruit cocktail-can/juice	cup	114	1.14	29.4	0.025	0	0.005	1.51
Kiwifruit-raw	item	46.4	0.752	11.3	0.334	0	0	2.58
Limes-raw	item	20.1	0.469	7.06	0.134	0	0.015	0.353
Melons-casaba-raw	cup	44.2	1.53	10.5	0.17	0	0	2

22

Food Name	Serving	KCAL Kc	PROT Gm	CARB Gm	FAT Gm	CHOL Mg	SAFA Gm	FIBD Gm
Nectarines-raw	item	66.6	1.28	16	0.626	0	-	2.18
Papaya nectar-can	cup	143	0.425	36.3	0.375	0	0.118	1.2
Pears-can/juice	cup	124	0.843	32.1	0.174	0	0.01	4.71
Pineapple-can/juice	cup	150	1.05	39.3	0.2	0	0.015	1.88
Pineapple juice-froz-dilu	cup	130	1	31.9	0.075	0	0.005	0.3
Pomegranates-raw	item	105	1.46	26.4	0.462	0	-	1.1
Strawberries-froz-unsweet	cup	52.2	0.641	13.6	0.164	0	0.009	3.9
Cranapple juice-can	cup	170	0.253	43.3	0	0	0	0
Fruit roll up-cherry	item	50	0	12	1	0	-	-
GRAINS								
Cornmeal-degerm-enr-cooked	cup	878	20.4	186	3.96	0	0.54	1.9
Macaroni-cooked-firm-hot	cup	183	6.2	36.9	0.871	0	0.124	2.08
Noodles-egg-enr-cooked	cup	200	7	37	2	50	-	3.52
Popcorn-popped-plain	cup	25	1	5	0	0	0	0.4
Popcorn-popped-sugar coat	cup	135	2	30	1	0	0.5	1.35
Pretzel-thin-stick	item	1.19	0.028	0.242	0.011	0	0	-
Rice-white-instant-hot	cup	162	3.4	35.1	0.264	0	0.073	1.32
Rice-white-long grain-cook	cup	264	5.51	57.2	0.574	0	0.158	2.13
Rice-white-parboil-cooked	cup	199	4.01	43.3	0.473	0	0.128	0.875
Spaghetti-cook-tender-hot	cup	155	5	32	1	0	-	2.24
Flour-wheat-enr-sifted	cup	419	11.9	87.7	1.12	0	0.178	3.11
Corn chips	ounce	155	1.7	16.9	9.14	0	1.5	1.66
Taco shells	item	49.8	0.967	7.24	2.15	0	-	0.88
Tortilla-corn	item	67.2	2.15	12.8	1.14	0	-	1.56

Food Name	Serving	KCAL Kc	PROT Gm	CARB Gm	FAT Gm	CHOL Mg	SAFA Gm	FIBD Gm
Rice-brown-Uncle Ben's	cup	220	5	46.4	1.82	0	0.462	2.48
Shake'n bake	ounce	116	2.44	17.7	4.26	-	-	-
Bisquick mix-dry	cup	480	8	76	16	-	-	3.02
Tortilla chips-Doritos	ounce	139	2	18.6	6.6	0	1.43	1.85
Croutons-herb seasoned	cup	100	4.29	20	0	0	0	1.41
Tortilla-flour	item	95	2.5	17.3	1.8	0	-	0.778
Rice-Spanish-home recipe	cup	213	4.4	40.7	4.2	0	-	1.83
Stuffing-mix-dry form	cup	111	3.9	21.7	1.1	-	-	-
Stuffing-mix-prepared	cup	501	9.1	49.8	30.5	-	-	-
Rice cake-regular	item	35	0.7	7.6	0.28	0	-	0.158
Noodles-Ramen-oriental	cup	207	5.9	30.7	8.6	-	-	2.04

MEATS

Food Name	Serving	KCAL Kc	PROT Gm	CARB Gm	FAT Gm	CHOL Mg	SAFA Gm	FIBD Gm
Bacon-pork-broiled/fried	slice	36.3	1.92	0.037	3.1	5.36	1.1	0
Roast beef-rib-lean/fat	slice	308	18.3	0	25.5	73.1	10.8	0
Roast beef-rib-lean	slice	122	13.9	0	7.03	41.3	2.96	0
Steak-sirloin-lean/fat	item	238	23.3	0	15.3	76.5	6.38	0
Steak-sirloin-lean/broiled	item	116	17	0	4.89	49.8	2	0
Steak-round-lean/fat	slice	179	26.2	0	7.5	72	2.8	0
Corned beef hash-canned	cup	400	19	24	25	50	11.9	-
Lamb-chop-lean/fat-broiled	serving	307	18.8	0	25.2	84.2	10.8	0
Lamb-chop/rib-lean-broiled	serving	134	15.8	0	7.38	51.9	2.65	0
Lamb-leg-lean/fat-roasted	slice	219	21.7	0	14	79	5.85	0
Beef-liver-fried/marg	slice	184	22.7	6.67	6.8	410	2.4	0
Ham-reg-roasted-pork	cup	249	31.7	0	12.6	82.6	4.37	0

Food Name	Serving	KCAL Kc	PROT Gm	CARB Gm	FAT Gm	CHOL Mg	SAFA Gm	FIBD Gm
Ham-reg-lunch meat-11% fat	slice	52	4.98	0.88	3	16.2	0.962	0
Pork-chop-lean/fat-broiled	item	284	19.3	0	22.3	77	8.06	0
Pork-chop-lean-broiled	item	169	18.4	0	10.1	63	3.48	0
Pork-loin-lean/fat-roast	item	268	22.4	0	19.1	80	6.92	0
Pork-loin-lean-roasted	slice	173	20.5	0	9.42	65.5	3.25	0
Pork-tenderloin-lean-roast	ounce	47.1	8.18	0	1.37	26.3	0.471	0
Bologna-pork	slice	56.8	3.52	0.168	4.57	13.6	1.58	0
Braunschweiger-saus-pork	slice	64.6	2.43	0.56	5.78	28.1	1.96	0
Sausage-patty-pork-cooked	item	100	5.31	0.28	8.41	22.4	2.92	0
Deviled ham-canned	tbsp	45	2	0	4	10	1.5	0
Frankfurter-hot dog-no bun	item	183	6.43	1.46	16.6	28.5	6.13	0
Sausage-link-pork-cooked	item	48	2.55	0.13	4.05	10.8	1.41	0
Salami-dry or hard-park	slice	40.7	2.26	0.16	3.37	7.9	1.19	0
Salami-cooked-beef	slice	60.3	3.46	0.646	4.76	15	2.07	0
Italian sausage-pork-link	item	216	13.4	1.01	17.2	52	6.05	0
Canadian bacon-pork-grill	slice	43	5.64	0.315	1.96	13.5	0.66	0
Livenwurst/liver saus-pork	slice	59	2.54	0.4	5.14	28	1.91	0
Polish sausage-pork	item	740	32	3.71	65.2	159	23.4	0
Kielbasa-pork/beef	slice	80.6	3.45	0.56	7.06	17.4	2.58	0
Knockwurst-pork/beef-link	item	209	8.08	1.2	18.9	39.4	6.94	0
Mortadella-pork/beef	slice	46.7	2.46	0.458	3.81	8.4	1.43	0
Bacon bits	tbsp	26.6	1.92	1.72	1.55	0	-	-
Spareribs-pork-braised	ounce	113	8.25	0	8.61	34.4	3.34	0
Steak-chicken fried	item	389	17.9	12.3	30	-	-	0
Pot roast-arm-beef-cooked	slice	231	33	0	9.98	101	3.79	0
Steak-rib-cooked	item	221	28	0	11.2	80	.75	0

Food Name	Serving	KCAL Kc	PROT Gm	CARB Gm	FAT Gm	CHOL Mg	SAFA Gm	FIBD Gm
Hamburger-ground-reg-baked	serving	244	19.6	0	17.8	74	6.99	0
Hamburger-ground-reg-fried	serving	260	20.3	0	19.2	75.7	7.53	0
MISCELLANEOUS								
Pickle/hot dog relish	ounce	35	0	8	0	0	0	-
Pickle/hamburger relish	ounce	30	0	7	0	0	0	-
Baking powder-home use	tsp	3.87	0.003	0.936	0	0	0	-
Baking powder-low sodium	tsp	7.4	0.004	1.79	0	0	0	-
Gelatin-dry envelope	item	25	6	0	0	0	0	0
Gelatin dessert-prep	cup	140	4	34	0	0	0	0
Olives-green-pickled-can	item	3.75	0.1	0.1	0.5	0	0.05	0.104
Olives-mission-rice-can	item	5	0.1	0.1	0.667	0	0.067	0.09
Pickle-dill-cucumber-med	item	5	0	1	0	0	0	0.78
Pickle-fresh pack-cucumber	item	5	0	1.5	0	0	0	0.09
Pickle-sweet-gherkin-small	item	20	0	5	0	0	0	0.165
Pickle relish-sweet	tbsp	20	0	5	0	0	0	-
Popsickle	item	70	0	18	0	0	0	-
Vinegar-cider	tbsp	0	0	1	0	0	0	0
Yeast-baker-dry-act-packet	serving	20	3	3	0	0	0	2.21
Yeast-brewers-dry	tbsp	25	3	3	0	0	0	-
Baking soda	tsp	0	0	0	0	0	0	0
Jello-gel-sugar free-prep	cup	16	2	0	0	0	0	0
Gel-D Zerta-low-cal-prep	cup	16	4	0	0	0	0	0
Chewing gum-Wrigleys	item	10	0	2.3	-	0	0	-

Food Name	Serving	KCAL Kc	PROT Gm	CARB Gm	FAT Gm	CHOL Mg	SAFA Gm	FIBD Gm
Vinegar-distilled	cup	29	0	12	0	0	0	0
Chewing gum-candy coated	item	5	-	1.6	-	0	0	-
NUTS/SEEDS								
Nuts-almond-shelled-sliver	cup	677	22.9	23.5	60	0	5.69	10.7
Nuts-brazil-dried-shelled	cup	918	20.1	17.9	92.7	0	22.6	10.8
Nuts-filbert-hazel-dri-chop	cup	727	15	17.6	72	0	5.29	9.77
Nuts-peanuts-oil roasted	cup	837	37.9	27.3	71	0	9.85	12.8
Peanut butter-smooth type	tbsp	94.1	3.94	3.32	8	0	1.53	0.96
Nuts-pecans-dried-halves	cup	720	8.37	19.7	73.1	0	5.85	7.02
Nuts-walnut-black-dri-chop	cup	759	30.4	15.1	70.7	0	4.54	8.08
Nuts-walnut-Persian/English	cup	770	17.2	22	74.2	0	6.7	5.76
Nuts-cashew-dry roasted	cup	786	21	44.8	63.5	0	12.5	10
Nuts-macadamia-dried	cup	941	11.1	18.4	98.8	0	14.8	12.4
Nuts-mixed-dry roasted	cup	814	23.7	34.7	70.5	0	9.45	11.6
Nuts-mixed-oil roasted	cup	876	23.8	30.4	80	0	12.4	12.8
Nuts-peanuts-Spanish-dried	cup	828	37.7	23.6	71.9	0	9.98	11.7
Nuts-pecans-oil roasted	cup	754	7.65	17.7	78.3	0	6.27	8.47
Nuts-pistachio-dried	cup	739	26.3	31.8	61.9	0	7.84	13.8
Nuts-pistachio-dry roasted	cup	776	19.1	35.2	67.6	0	8.56	13.8
Seeds-pumpkin/squash-roast	cup	285	11.9	34.4	12.4	0	2.35	29.4
Seeds-sesame-roasted-whole	ounce	161	4.82	7.31	13.6	0	1.91	5.32
Seeds-sunflower-oil roast	cup	830	28.8	19.9	77.6	0	8.13	9.18
Peanut butter-low sodium	tbsp	95	5	2.5	8.5	0	1.36	1.7
Nuts-peanuts-oil-salted	cup	837	37.9	27.3	71	0	9.85	12.8

Food Name	Serving	KCAL Kc	PROT Gm	CARB Gm	FAT Gm	CHOL Mg	SAFA Gm	FIBD Gm
Peanut butter-chunk style	tbsp	94.8	3.87	3.48	8.04	0	1.54	1.06
Peanut butter-old fashion	tbsp	95	4.2	2.7	8.1	0	1.5	1.06

POULTRY PRODUCTS

Food Name	Serving	KCAL Kc	PROT Gm	CARB Gm	FAT Gm	CHOL Mg	SAFA Gm	FIBD Gm
Chicken-breast-fried/flour	item	436	62.4	3.22	17.4	176	4.8	0.07
Chicken-drumstick-fried	item	120	13.2	0.8	6.72	44	1.79	0
Chicken-breast-fri/batter	item	728	69.6	25.2	36.9	238	9.86	-
Turkey-dark meat-no skin	cup	262	40	0	10.1	119	3.39	0
Turkey-light-no skin-roast	cup	219	41.9	0	4.5	97	1.44	0
Turkey-light/dark-no skin	cup	238	41	0	6.95	107	2.29	0
Turk-breast-no skin-roast	item	826	184	0	4.5	508	1.47	0
Chicken-giblets-fri/flour	cup	402	47.2	6.31	19.5	647	5.5	-
Chicken-giblets-simmered	cup	228	37.5	1.37	6.92	570	2.16	0
Chicken-liver-simmered	cup	219	34.1	1.23	7.63	883	2.58	0
Chicken-breast-roasted	item	386	58.4	0	15.3	166	4.3	0
Chicken-breast-stewed	item	404	60.3	0	16.3	166	4.58	0
Chicken-breast-no skin-fri	item	322	57.5	0.88	8.1	156	2.22	0
Chick-breast-no skin-roast	item	284	53.4	0	6.14	146	1.74	0
Chicken-leg-roasted	item	265	29.6	0	15.4	105	4.24	0
Chicken-leg-no skin-roast	item	182	25.7	0	8.01	89	2.18	0
Chicken-leg-no skin-stewed	item	187	26.5	0	8.14	90	2.22	0
Chicken-thigh-fried/flour	item	162	16.6	1.97	9.29	60	2.54	0.04
Chicken-thigh-no skin-roast	item	109	13.5	0	5.66	49	1.57	0
Chicken-wing-fried/flour	item	103	8.36	0.76	7.09	26	1.94	0
Chicken-wing-roasted	item	99	9.13	0	6.62	29	1.85	0

Food Name	Serving	KCAL Kc	PROT Gm	CARB Gm	FAT Gm	CHOL Mg	SAFA Gm	FIBD Gm
Chicken-wing-stewed	item	100	9.11	0	6.73	28	1.88	0
Duck-flesh & skin-roasted	item	2574	145	0	217	640	73.9	0
Duck-no skin-roasted	item	890	104	0	49.5	396	18.4	0
Chicken-frankfurter	item	116	5.82	3.06	8.76	45.5	2.49	0.01
Chicken-liver pate-can	tbsp	26	1.75	0.85	1.7	-	-	0
Chicken roll-light	slice	45	5.54	0.695	2.09	14.2	0.574	-
Chicken spread-canned	tbsp	25	2	0.7	1.52	-	-	-
Turk ham-cured thigh meat	slice	36.5	5.37	0.105	1.44	15.9	0.483	0
Turkey loaf-breast	serving	31.2	6.39	0	0.449	11.6	0.136	0
Turkey pastrami	slice	40	5.21	0.47	1.76	15.3	0.514	0
Turkey roll-light	ounce	41.7	5.31	0.15	2.05	12.2	0.574	0
SAUCES/DIPS								
Sauce-chili-bottled	tbsp	16	0.4	3.7	0	0	0	-
Sauce-Heinz 57	tbsp	15	0.4	2.7	0.2	0	0	-
Sauce-tartar-regular	tbsp	75	0	1	8	9	1.5	-
Dip-guacamole-Kraft	tbsp	25	0.5	1.5	2	0	-	-
Dip-French onion-Kraft	tbsp	30	0.5	1.5	2	0	-	-
Sauce-taco-canned	fl oz	11	0.4	2.2	0.7	0	0	-
Sauce-salsa/chilies-canned	fl oz	10	0.4	2	0.7	0	0	-
Sauce-picante-canned	fl oz	9	0.3	1.9	0.5	0	0	-
Tomato catsup	tbsp	15	0	4	0	0	0	-
Sauce-barbecue	cup	188	4.5	32	4.5	0	0.675	2.3
Mustard-yellow-prepared	tsp	5	0.1	0.1	0.1	0	0	0.06

Food Name	Serving	KCAL Kc	PROT Gm	CARB Gm	FAT Gm	CHOL Mg	SAFA Gm	FIBD Gm
Sauce-bearnaise-mix/milk	cup	701	8.34	17.5	68.3	189	41.8	0.09
Sauce-cheese-mix/milk	cup	307	16	23.2	17.1	53	9.32	0.1
Sauce-curry-mix/milk	cup	269	10.7	25.7	14.7	35.4	6.04	0.9
Sauce-mushroom-mix/milk	cup	227	11.3	23.8	10.3	34	5.39	0.5
Sauce-sweet/sour-mix/prep	cup	294	0.751	72.7	0.063	0	0	-
Sauce-soy	tbsp	9.54	0.931	1.53	0.014	0	0.002	-
Gravy-beef-canned	cup	123	8.74	11.2	5.49	6.99	2.69	0.093
Gravy-chicken-canned	cup	188	4.59	12.9	13.6	4.76	3.36	-
Gravy-turkey-canned	cup	121	6.2	12.2	5.01	4.76	1.48	-
Sauce-marinara-canned	cup	170	4	25.5	8.38	0	1.2	-
Sauce-tomato-can-salt add	cup	73.5	3.26	17.6	0.417	0	0.059	3.68
Sauce-tomato-Spanish-can	cup	80.5	3.51	17.7	0.659	0	0.092	3.66
Sauce-spaghetti-canned	cup	271	4.53	39.7	11.9	0	1.7	-
Sauce-sour cream-mix/milk	cup	509	19.1	45.4	30.2	91	16.1	-
Sauce-teriyaki-bottled	tbsp	15.1	1.07	2.87	0	0	0	-
Horseradish-prepared	tbsp	6	0.2	1.4	0	0	0	-
Sauce-worcestershire	tbsp	12	0.3	2.7	0	0	0	-
Sauce-tabasco	tsp	0	0.1	0.1	0	0	0	0
Mustard-brown-prepared	cup	228	14.8	13.3	15.8	0	-	-
Sauce-tomato-can-low sod	cup	90	4	18	0	0	0	3.39
SOUPS								
Soup-cream/chick-can-milk	cup	191	7.46	15	11.5	27.3	4.64	0.5
Soup-cream/mushroom-milk	cup	203	6.05	15	13.6	19.8	5.13	-
Soup-tomato-can-milk	cup	161	6.1	22.3	6	17.4	2.9	0.8

30

Food Name	Serving	KCAL Kc	PROT Gm	CARB Gm	FAT Gm	CHOL Mg	SAFA Gm	FBD Gm
Soup-bean/bacon-can-water	cup	173	7.89	22.8	5.94	2.53	1.52	3.2
Soup-beef broth-can-ready	cup	16.8	2.74	0.096	0.528		0.264	0
Soup-clam-Manhattan-water	cup	78.1	2.2	12.2	2.22	2.44	0.383	0
Soup-minestrome-can-water	cup	81.9	4.26	11.2	2.51	2.41	0.554	1.9
Soup-pea-split-can-water	cup	189	10.3	28	4.4	7.59	1.77	-
Soup-tomato-can-water	cup	85.4	2.05	16.6	1.92	0	0.366	0.9
Soup-vegetable beef-can	cup	78.4	5.61	10.2	1.91	4.9	0.858	0.98
Soup-vegetarian-can-water	cup	72	2.1	12	1.93	0	0.289	1.21
Soup-beef broth-dehy-cubed	item	6.12	0.62	0.58	0.14	0.144	0.072	-
Soup-onion-dehy-packet	serving	115	4.52	20.9	2.33	1.95	0.538	2.2
Soup-cream/celery-can-milk	cup	164	5.68	14.5	9.7	32.2	3.94	0.77
Soup-cheese-can-milk	cup	230	9.46	16.2	14.6	47.7	9.11	-
Soup-chick broth-can/water	cup	39	4.93	0.93	1.39	0	0.39	0
Soup-chicken noodle-can	cup	74.7	4.05	9.35	2.46	7.23	0.65	1.45
Soup-clam-New England-milk	cup	163	9.47	16.6	6.6	22.3	2.95	-
Soup-cream/potato-can-water	cup	148	5.78	17.2	6.45	22.3	3.77	-
Soup-black bean-can-water	cup	116	5.63	19.8	1.51	0	0.395	-
Soup-beef-chunky-can	cup	170	11.7	19.6	5.14	14.4	2.55	-
Soup-chicken-chunky-can	cup	178	12.7	17.3	6.63	30.1	1.98	-
Soup-chicken/rice-can	cup	127	12.3	13	3.19	12	0.96	1.44
Soup-onion-can-water	cup	57.8	3.75	8.17	1.74	0	0.265	-
Soup-pea-green-can-water	cup	165	8.6	26.5	2.94	0	1.4	-
Soup-tomato rice-can-water	cup	119	2.11	21.9	2.72	2.47	0.519	1.7
Soup-turkey-chunky-can	cup	135	10.2	14.1	4.41	9.44	1.23	2.5
Soup-turkey noodle-can	cup	68.3	3.9	8.63	1.99	4.88	0.561	0.7
Soup-turkey vegetable-can	cup	72.3	3.09	8.63	3.04	2.41	0.892	0.964

Food Name	Serving	KCAL Kc	PROT Gm	CARB Gm	FAT Gm	CHOL Mg	SAFA Gm	FIBD Gm
SUGARS/SWEETS								
Nuts-coconut-dri-flake-can	cup	341	2.58	31.5	24.4	0	21.6	4.4
Icing-cake-white-boiled	cup	295	1	75	0	0	0	0
Icing-cake-white/coco-boil	cup	605	3	124	13	0	11	-
Icing-cake-choc-mix/prep	cup	1035	9	185	38	0	23.4	0-
Icing-cake-fudge-mix/water	cup	830	7	183	16	0	5.1	-
Icing-cake-white-uncooked	cup	1200	2	260	231	0	12.7	-
Candy-caramels-plan/choc	ounce	115	1	22	3	0	1.6	0.784
Candy-milk chocolate-plain	ounce	145	2	16	9	0	5.5	-
Candy-chocolate-semisweet	cup	860	7	97	61	0	36.2	-
Candy-choc coated peanuts	ounce	160	5	11	12	0	4	-
Candy-fondant-uncoated	ounce	105	0	25	1	0	0.1	0
Candy-fudge-choc-plain	ounce	115	1	21	3	0	1.3	-
Candy-gum drops	ounce	00	0	25	0	0	0	0
Candy-hard	ounce	110	0	28	0	0	0	0
Marshmallows	ounce	90	1	23	0	0	0	0
Honey-strained/estracted	tbsp	65	0	17	0	0	0	0.06
Jams/preserves-regular	tbsp	55	0	14	0	0	0	0.2
Molasses-cane-light	tbsp	50	0	13	-	0	-	0
Molasses-cane-blackstrap	tbsp	45	0	11	-	0	-	0
Sugar-brown-pressed down	cup	820	0	212	0	0	0	0
Sugar-white-granulated	tbsp	45	0	12	0	0	0	0
Sugar-white-powder-sifted	cup	385	0	100	0	0	0	0
Nuts-coconut-dried-shred	cup	466	2.68	44.3	33	0	29.3	3.9
Nuts-coconut cream-raw	cup	792	8.7	16	83.2	0	73.8	1.6

32

Food Name	Serving	KCAL Kc	PROT Gm	CARB Gm	FAT Gm	CHOL Mg	SAFA Gm	FIBD Gm
Candy-milk choc/peanuts	ounce	154	4	12.6	10.8	-	5.22	-
Candy-milk choc/almonds	ounce	151	2.6	14.5	10.1	-	4.06	-
Sugar-Sweet & Low-packet	item	4	-	0.9	-	0	-	-
Sugar-Equal-packet	item	4	0	1	0	0	0	-
Candy-Life Savers	item	7.8	0	1.94	0.02	0	0	0
Candy- M & M's-package	item	220	3	31	10	-	4.73	-
Candy-Snickers bar	item	270	6	33	13	-	5.05	-
Candy-Milky Way bar	item	260	3	43	9	-	5.6	-
Candy-Kit Kat bar	item	210	3	25	11	-	-	-
Candy-Bit O Honey	ounce	121	0.9	21.2	3.6	-	1.85	-
Candy-Almond Joy	ounce	151	1.7	18.5	7.8	-	1.74	-
Candy-jelly beans	item	6.6	0	2.64	0	0	0	0
Candy-peanut brittle	ounce	123	2.4	20.4	4.4	-	1.85	-
Candy-peanut butter cup	piece	92	2.2	8.7	5.35	2.5	2.8	-
Candy-lollipop	item	108	0	28	0	0	0	0
VEGETABLES								
V-8 veg juice-low sodium	cup	51	0	9.72	0	0	0	2.7
Tomato juice-low sodium	cup	41.5	1.85	10.3	0.146	0	0.02	2.8
Beans-garbanzo-can	serving	27.8	1.31	4.66	0.511	0	0.07	1.4
Beans-navy pea-dry cooked	cup	225	15	40	1	0	-	9.31
Beans-red kidney-can	cup	230	15	42	1	0	-	12.5
Peas-split-dry-cooked	cup	230	16	42	1	0	-	10.5
Asparagus-froz-boil-spears	cup	50.4	5.31	8.77	0.756	0	0.171	2.16
Beans-lima-froz-boil-drain	cup	170	10.3	32	0.578	0	0.131	8.33

Food Name	Serving	KCAL Kc	PROT Gm	CARB Gm	FAT Gm	CHOL Mg	SAFA Gm	FIBD Gm
Beans-snap-green-raw-boil	cup	43.8	2.36	9.86	0.35	0	0.08	2.25
Beans-green-froz-French	cup	35.1	1.84	8.26	0.189	0	0.041	2.16
Beans-snap-green-can-cuts	cup	27	1.55	6.08	0.135	0	0.03	1.76
Beans-snap-wax-raw-boil	cup	43.8	2.36	9.86	0.35	0	0.08	2.25
Beans-snap-yellow/wax-can	cup	27.2	1.56	6.12	0.136	0	0.03	1.77
Beans-mung-sprouted-boil	cup	26.3	2.54	5.24	0.113	0	0.031	2.7
Beets-can-sliced-drain	cup	52.7	1.55	12.2	0.238	0	0.039	2.89
Cowpeas-blackeye-raw-boil	cup	160	5.23	33.5	0.627	0	0.158	11
Cowpeas-blackeye-froz-boil	cup	224	14.4	40.4	1.12	0	0.298	9.8
Broccoli-raw	cup	24.6	2.62	4.61	0.308	0	0.048	2.46
Broccoli-raw-boil-drain	cup	43.4	4.62	7.84	0.543	0	0.084	4.03
Cabbage-white mustard-raw	cup	9.1	1.05	1.53	0.14	0	0.018	0.7
Broccoli-froz-boil-drain	cup	51.8	5.74	9.85	0.21	0	0.033	7.3
Cabbage-common-raw-shred	cup	21.6	1.09	4.83	0.162	0	0.021	1.8
Cabbage-common-boil-drain	cup	30.5	1.39	6.92	0.363	0	0.046	4
Cabbage-red-raw-shredded	cup	18.9	0.973	4.28	0.182	0	0.024	1.4
Cabbage-celery-raw	cup	12.2	0.912	2.45	0.152	0	0.033	0.76
Cabbage-white mustard-boil	cup	20.4	2.65	3.03	0.272	0	0.036	2.72
Carrot-raw-whole-scraped	item	31	0.74	7.3	0.137	0	0.022	2.3
Carrot-raw-shred-scraped	cup	47.3	1.13	11.2	0.209	0	0.033	3.52
Carrots-boil-drain-sliced	cup	70.2	1.7	16.3	0.28	0	0.053	5.77
Carrots-can-sliced-drain	cup	33.6	0.934	8.08	0.277	0	0.052	2.19
Cauliflower-raw-chopped	cup	24	1.99	4.92	0.18	0	0.027	2.4
Cauliflower-raw-boil-drain	cup	30	2.32	5.74	0.22	0	0.046	2.73
Cauliflower-froz-boil	cup	34.2	2.9	6.75	0.396	0	0.059	3.24
Celery-pascal-raw-stalk	item	6.4	0.3	1.46	0.056	0	0.015	0.64

34

Food Name	Serving	KCAL Kc	PROT Gm	CARB Gm	FAT Gm	CHOL Mg	SAFA Gm	FIBD Gm
Celery-pascal-raw-diced	cup	19.2	0.9	4.38	0.168	0	0.044	1.92
Collards-raw-boil-drain	cup	34.6	1.73	7.85	0.243	0	-	2.1
Collards-frozen-boil-drain	cup	61.2	5.05	12.1	0.697	0	-	5.2
Corn-kernels from 1 ear	item	83.2	2.56	19.3	0.986	0	0.152	2.85
Corn-kernels & cob-froz-boil	item	117	3.92	28.1	0.932	0	0.144	2.65
Corn-froz-boil-kernels	cup	134	4.98	33.9	0.116	0	0.018	3.47
Corn-sweet-cream style-can	cup	184	4.45	46.4	1.08	0	0.166	3.07
Corn-sweet-can-drained	cup	134	4.32	30.7	1.65	0	0.254	2.31
Cucumber-raw-sliced	cup	13.5	0.562	3.03	0.135	0	0.034	1.04
Endive-raw-chopped	cup	8.5	0.625	1.68	0.1	0	0.024	-
Lettuce-butterhead-leaves	slice	1.95	0.194	0.348	0.03	0	0.004	0.15
Lettuce-iceberg-raw-leaves	piece	2.61	0.202	0.418	0.038	0	0.005	0.2
Lettuce-iceberg-raw-chop	cup	7.15	0.556	1.15	0.105	0	0.014	0.55
Lettuce-looseleaf-raw	cup	9.9	0.715	1.93	0.165	0	0.022	0.76
Mushrooms-raw-chopped	cup	17.5	1.46	3.26	0.294	0	0.039	0.91
Onions-mature-raw-chopped	cup	60.8	1.86	13.8	0.256	0	0.042	2.56
Carrots-frozen-boil-drain	cup	52.6	1.74	12	0.161	0	0.031	5.4
Onions-mature-boil-drain	cup	92.4	2.86	21.3	0.399	0	0.065	1.68
Onions-young green	item	1.25	0.087	0.278	0.007	0	0.001	0.12
Parsley-raw-chopped	tbsp	1.32	0.088	0.276	0.03	0	0.005	0.176
Peas-green-can-drained	cup	117	7.51	21.4	0.595	0	0.105	5.78
Peas-green-froz-boil-drain	cup	125	8.24	22.8	0.432	0	0.078	6.08
Peppers-hot-red-dried	tsp	5	0	1	0	0		0.685
Potato-French fried-raw	item	13.5	0.2	1.8	0.7	0	0.17	0.16
Potato-French fried-froz	item	11.1	0.173	1.7	0.438	0	0.208	0.16
Potato-hashed brown-froz	cup	340	4.93	43.8	17.9	0	7.01	1.5

Food Name	Serving	KCAL Kc	PROT Gm	CARB Gm	FAT Gm	CHOL Mg	SAFA Gm	FIBD Gm
Potato-mashed-milk/butter	cup	223	3.95	35.1	8.88	4.2	2.17	3.15
Potato-mashed-dehy-prep	cup	166	4.2	27.5	4.62	4	1.43	1.2
Potato chips-salt added	item	10.5	0.128	1.04	0.708	0	0.181	0.029
Radishes-raw	item	0.765	0.027	0.162	0.024	0	0.001	0.1
Sauerkraut-canned	cup	44.8	2.15	10.1	0.33	0	0.083	6.06
Spinach-raw-chopped	cup	12.3	1.6	1.96	0.196	0	0.032	1.46
Spinach-boil-drain	cup	41.4	5.35	6.75	0.468	0	0.076	3.96
Spinach-froz-boil-chopped	cup	57.4	6.44	10.9	0.431	0	0.068	4.51
Squash-summer-boil-sliced	cup	36	1.64	7.76	0.558	0	0.115	2.52
Squash-winter-bake-mash	cup	80	1.82	17.9	1.29	0	0.267	5.74
Sweet potato-bake-peel	item	117	1.96	27.7	0.125	0	0.027	3.42
Sweet potato-boil-mashed	cup	344	5.41	79.6	0.984	0	0.21	9.84
Sweet potato-candied	piece	144	0.914	29.3	3.41	0	1.42	1.1
Sweet potato-can-mashed	cup	258	5.05	59.2	0.51	0	0.11	4.59
Tomato-red-ripe	item	25.8	1.05	5.71	0.406	0	0.056	1.6
Tomato-red-can-whole	cup	48	2.23	10.3	0.576	0	0.084	1.93
Tomato juice-can	cup	41.5	1.85	10.3	0.146	0	0.02	2.9
Tomato powder	ounce	85.8	3.67	21.2	0.125	0	0.018	-
Alfalfa seeds-sprouted-raw	cup	9.57	1.32	1.25	0.228	0	0.023	0.726
Artichokes-boil-drain	item	60	4.18	13.4	0.192	0	0.044	4
Beans-lima-can	cup	186	11.3	34.4	0.744	0	0.168	10.4
Beans-pinto-froz-boil	ounce	46	2.64	8.77	0.136	0	0.016	1.39
Beans-shellie-can	cup	73.5	4.31	15.2	0.466	0	0.056	12
Chives-raw-chopped	tbsp	0.75	0.084	0.114	0.018	0	0.003	0.096
Eggplant-boiled-drained	cup	26.9	0.8	6.37	0.221	0	0.042	2.69
Garlic-raw-cloves	item	4.47	0.191	0.992	0.015	0	0.003	-

Food Name	Serving	KCAL Kc	PROT Gm	CARB Gm	FAT Gm	CHOL Mg	SAFA Gm	FIBD Gm
Leeks-boil-drain	item	38.4	1.01	9.45	0.248	0	0.033	3.97
Mushrooms-boil-drain	item	3.24	0.26	0.617	0.056	0	0.007	0.264
Mushrooms-can-drain	item	2.88	0.224	0.595	0.035	0	0.005	0.216
Onion rings-froz-prep-heat	item	40.7	0.534	3.82	2.67	0	0.858	0.382
Peppers-jalapeno-can-chop	cup	32.6	1.09	0.664	0.816	0	0.084	-
Potato-skin-baked	item	115	2.49	26.7	0.058	0	0.015	3.02
Potato-au gratin-home rec	cup	323	12.4	27.6	18.6	56.4	11.6	4.41
Potato-hash brown-prep-raw	cup	239	3.77	11.6	21.7	-	8.48	3.12
Potato-scallop-home rec	cup	211	7.03	26.4	9.02	29.4	5.52	4.41
Potato-scallop-mix-prep	ounce	26.4	0.602	3.63	1.22	-	0.748	0.54
Potato pancakes-home rec	item	495	4.63	26.4	12.6	93.5	3.42	-
Pumpkin pie mix-can	cup	281	2.94	71.3	0.351	0	0.176	-
Rutabagas-boil-drain	cup	57.8	1.87	13.2	0.323	0	0.042	2.5
Seaweed-wakame-raw	ounce	12.8	0.861	2.6	0.182	0	0.037	1.2
Squash-zucchini-raw-sliced	cup	18.2	1.51	3.77	0.182	0	0.038	2
Squash-zucchini-raw-boil	cup	28.8	1.15	7.07	0.09	0	0.018	2.3
Squash-zucchini-froz-boil	cup	37.9	2.56	7.94	0.29	0	0.06	3.23
Squash-zucchini-italia-can	cup	65.8	2.34	15.5	0.25	0	0.052	7.02
Succotash-boil-drain	cup	221	9.73	46.8	1.54	0	0.284	14
Tomato-red-raw-boil	cup	64.8	2.57	14	0.984	0	0.137	2.1
Tomato-stew-cook-home rec	cup	79.8	1.98	13.2	2.71	0	0.526	1.04
Tomato-red-can-stewed	cup	66.3	2.37	16.5	0.357	0	0.051	2.04
Tomato-paste-can-low sod	cup	220	9.9	49.3	2.33	0	0.333	11.3
Tomato puree-can-low sod	cup	103	4.18	25.1	0.3	0	0.04	5.75
Vegetable juice-can	cup	46	1.52	11	0.218	0	0.032	2.7
Nuts-chestnuts-roasted	ounce	67.9	1.27	14.9	0.34	0	0.05	2.19

Food Name	Serving	KCAL Kc	PROT Gm	CARB Gm	FAT Gm	CHOL Mg	SAFA Gm	FIBD Gm
Squash-hubbard-boil-mash	cup	70.8	3.49	15.2	0.873	0	0.179	4.2
Squash-butternut-baked	cup	82	1.84	21.5	0.185	0	0.039	3.5
Squash-acorn-baked	cup	115	2.29	29.9	0.287	0	0.059	4.3
Lettuce-romaine-raw-shred	cup	8.96	0.9	1.33	0.112	0	0.014	0.952
Soybean-dry-cooked	cup	234	19.8	19.4	10.3	0	-	-
Tofu-soybean curd	piece	86	9.4	2.9	5	0	-	1.44
Tomato-can-low sodium diet	cup	48	2.23	10.3	0.576	0	0.084	1.69
Spinach-can-solids/liquids	cup	44.5	4.94	6.83	0.866	0	0.14	5.08
Tomato paste-can-salt add	cup	220	9.9	49.3	2.33	0	0.332	11.3
Tomato puree-can-salt add	cup	103	4.18	25.1	0.3	0	0.04	5.75
Miso-fermented soybeans	cup	567	32.5	76.9	16.7	0	2.41	9.9
Beans-baked beans-canned	cup	236	12.2	52.1	1.14	0	0.295	19.6
Beans-refried beans	cup	271	15.8	46.8	2.7	0	1.04	11.6

38

FAST FOOD TABLES

Food Name	Oz Gm	KCAL Gm	PROT Gm	CARB Gm	FIBD Gm	FAT Gm	SAFA Gm	CHOL Mg
Restaurant: Arby's								
Regular Roast Beef	5 147	353	22.2	31.6	1	14.8	7.3	39
Beef 'N Cheddar	7 197	455	25.7	27.7	1	26.8	7.6	63
Chicken Breast Sandwich	7 184	493	23.0	47.9	1	25.0	5.1	91
Roast Chicken Club	8 234	610	31.0	40.0	2	33.0	8.0	80
Turkey Deluxe	7 197	375	23.8	32.5	2	16.6	4.1	39
Ham 'N Cheese	6 156	292	22.9	19.2	1	13.7	4.7	45
Super Roast Beef	8 234	501	25.1	50.4	1	22.1	8.5	40
French Fries	3 71	246	2.1	29.8	2	13.2	3.0	0
Restaurant: Burger King								
Whopper/Everything	10 270	628	27.0	46.0	2	36.0	12.0	90
Whopper/Cheese	10 294	706	32.0	47.0	2	43.0	17.0	113
Hamburger	4 108	272	15.0	29.0	1	12.0	4.0	37
Cheeseburger	4 121	318	17.0	30.0	1	15.0	7.0	48
Bacon Double Chburger	6 160	515	33.0	27.0	1	31.0	15.0	104
Hamburger Deluxe	5 138	344	15.0	30.0	1	17.0	6.0	41
Cheeseburger Deluxe	5 151	390	17.0	31.0	2	20.0	8.0	52
Ocean Catch Filet	7 194	488	19.0	45.0	2	25.0	4.0	77
Chicken Specialty Sandwich	8 229	685	26.0	56.0	2	40.0	8.0	82
Chicken Tenders	3 90	236	20.0	10.0	1	10.0	2.0	47
French Fries	4 111	341	3.0	24.0	3	13.0	7.0	14
Onion Rings	3 86	302	4.0	28.0	2	16.0	3.0	0
Brkfast Cros/Bacon	4 118	355	14.0	20.0	1	24.0	8.0	249
Brkfast Cros/Sausage	6 159	538	20.0	20.0	1	40.0	13.0	293
Brkfast Cros/Ham/Egg/Ch	5 144	346	19.0	19.0	1	21.0	7.0	241

40

Food Name	Oz	Gm	KCAL Gm	PROT Gm	CARB Gm	FIBD Gm	FAT Gm	SAFA Gm	CHOL Mg
Brkfast Bagel Sand/Bacon	6	169	438	20.0	46.0	2	20.0	7.0	274
Brkfast Bagel Sand/ Sausage/Egg/Cheese	7	210	626	27.0	49.0	2	36.0	12.0	318
Brkfast Bagel Sand/Ham/ Egg/Cheese	7	196	418	23.0	46.0	2	15.0	6.0	287
Scrambled Egg Platter	7	211	549	17.0	44.0	3	30.0	9.0	370
Scrambled Egg Plat/Saus	9	260	768	26.0	47.0	3	53.0	15.0	412
Scrambled Egg Plat/Bacon	8	221	610	21.0	44.0	3	39.0	11.0	373
French Toast Sticks	5	141	538	10.0	53.0	3	32.0	5.0	80
Great Danish	3	71	500	5.0	40.0	0	36.0	23.0	6
Vanilla Shake	10	284	334	9.0	51.0	1	10.0	6.0	39
Chocolate Shake	10	284	326	9.0	49.0	2	10.0	6.0	33
Apple Pie	4	125	311	3.0	44.0	2	14.0	4.0	4
Chicken Salad	9	258	142	20.0	8.0	2	4.0	1.0	50
Chef Salad	10	273	178	17.0	7.0	2	9.0	4.0	120
Garden Salad	8	223	95	6.0	8.0	2	5.0	3.0	15
Side Salad	5	135	25	1.0	5.0	2	0.0	0.0	0
Resaurant: Dairy Queen									
Cone, Small	3	85	140	3.0	22.0	0	4.0	1.7	10
Cone, Regular	5	142	240	6.0	38.0	0	7.0	3.1	15
Cone, Large	8	213	340	9.0	57.0	0	10.0	5.2	25
Cone, Small, Choco-Dipped	3	92	190	3.0	25.0	2	9.0	4.2	10
Cone, Reg, Choco-Dipped	6	156	340	6.0	42.0	3	16.0	7.8	20
Cone, Lg, Choco-Dipped	8	234	510	9.0	64.0	4	24.0	11.8	30
Chocolate Sundae, Small	4	106	190	3.0	33.0	1	4.0	2.2	10

Food Name	Oz	Gm	KCAL Gm	PROT Gm	CARB Gm	FIBD Gm	FAT Gm	SAFA Gm	CHOL Mg
Chocolate Sundae, Regular	6	177	310	5.0	56.0	1	8.0	3.8	20
Chocolate Sundae, Large	9	248	440	8.0	78.0	2	10.0	5.6	30
Chocolate Shake, Small	9	241	409	8.0	69.0	1	11.0	7.8	30
Chocolate Shake, Regular	15	418	710	14.0	120.0	2	19.0	12.4	50
Chocolate Shake, Large	17	489	831	16.0	140.0	2	22.0	14.2	60
Chocolate Malt, Small	9	241	438	8.0	77.0	2	10.0	6.5	30
Chocolate Malt, Regular	15	418	760	14.0	134.0	3	18.0	11.2	50
Chocolate Malt, Large	17	489	889	16.0	157.0	3	21.0	13.1	60
Float	14	397	410	5.0	82.0	3	7.0	3.5	20
Peanut Buster Parfait	11	305	740	16.0	94.0	6	34.0	14.1	30
Parfait	10	283	430	8.0	76.0	1	8.0	5.8	30
Freeze	14	397	500	9.0	89.0	0	12.0	7.0	30
Mr Misty, Small	9	248	190	0.0	48.0	0	0.0	0.0	0
Mr Misty, Regular	12	330	250	0.0	63.0	0	0.0	0.0	0
Mr. Misty, Large	16	439	340	0.0	84.0	0	0.0	0.0	0
Mr Misty Kiss	3	89	70	0.0	17.0	0	0.0	0.0	0
Mr Misty Freeze	15	411	500	9.0	91.0	0	12.0	7.0	30
Mr Misty Float	15	411	390	5.0	74.0	0	7.0	3.5	20
Buster Bar	5	149	448	10.0	41.0	6	29.0	8.9	10
Fudge Nut Bar	5	142	406	8.0	40.0	2	25.0	11.3	10
Dilly Bar	3	85	210	3.0	21.0	1	13.0	11.1	10
DQ Sandwich	2	60	140	3.0	24.0	0	4.0	2.0	5
Chipper Sandwich	4	113	318	5.0	56.0	0	7.0	5.7	13
Heath Blizzard, Regular	14	404	800	15.0	125.0	3	24.0	13.8	65
Single Hamburger	5	148	360	21.0	33.0	1	16.0	5.7	45

Food Name	Oz	Gm	KCAL Gm	PROT Gm	CARB Gm	FIBD Gm	FAT Gm	SAFA Gm	CHOL Mg
Double Hamburger	7	210	530	36.0	33.0	1	28.0	10.6	85
Triple Hamburger	10	272	710	51.0	33.0	1	45.0	15.4	135
Single Hamburger/Cheese	6	162	410	24.0	33.0	1	20.0	8.5	50
Double Hamburger/Cheese	8	239	650	43.0	34.0	1	37.0	16.1	95
Triple Hamburger/Cheese	11	301	820	58.0	34.0	1	50.0	21.0	145
Hot Dog	4	100	280	11.0	21.0	1	16.0	6.7	45
Hot Dog/Chili	5	128	320	13.0	23.0	1	20.0	7.4	55
Hot Dog/Cheese	4	114	330	15.0	21.0	1	21.0	9.4	55
Super Hot Dog	6	175	520	17.0	44.0	1	27.0	10.2	80
Super Hot Dog/Chili	8	218	570	21.0	47.0	2	32.0	11.8	100
Super Hot Dog/Cheese	7	196	580	22.0	45.0	1	34.0	14.4	100
Fish Filet	6	177	430	20.0	45.0	1	18.0	5.4	40
Fish Filet/Cheese	7	191	483	23.0	46.0	1	22.0	9.4	49
Chicken Breast Filet	7	202	608	27.0	46.0	2	34.0	8.4	78
Chicken Breast Filet/Cheese	8	216	661	30.0	47.0	2	38.0	12.2	87
All White Chicken Nuggets	4	276	276	16.0	13.0	1	18.0	6.1	39
French Fries, Small	3	71	200	2.0	25.0	2	10.0	4.4	10
French Fries, Large	4	113	320	3.0	40.0	3	16.0	7.1	15
Onion Rings	3	85	280	4.0	31.0	3	16.0	6.7	15
Restaurant: Domino's Pizza (2 slices of each pizza)									
Cheese Pizza	6	168	376	21.6	56.3	6	10.0	5.5	19
Pepperoni Pizza	7	187	460	24.1	55.6	5	17.5	8.4	28
Sausage/Mushroom Pizza	7	200	430	24.2	55.3	8	15.8	7.7	28
Veggie Pizza	9	261	498	31.0	60.0	8	18.5	10.2	36
Deluxe Pizza	8	234	498	26.7	59.2	7	20.4	9.3	40

43

Food Name	Oz	Gm	KCAL Gm	PROT Gm	CARB Gm	FIBD Gm	FAT Gm	SAFA Gm	CHOL Mg
Dble Chs/Pepperoni Pizza	8	227	545	32.1	55.2	8	25.3	13.3	48
Ham Pizza	7	186	417	23.2	58.0	2	11.0	5.9	26
Restaurant: Kentucky Fried Chicken									
Nuggets	1	16	46	2.8	2.2	0	2.9	0.7	12
Chicken Littles Sandwich	2	47	169	5.7	13.8	0	10.1	2.0	18
Buttermilk Biscuit	2	65	235	4.5	28.0	1	11.9	3.2	1
Mashed Potatoes/Gravy	4	98	71	2.4	11.9	1	1.6	1.6	0
French Fries, Regular	3	77	244	3.2	31.1	2	11.9	2.6	2
Corn-on-the-cob	5	143	176	5.1	31.9	7	3.1	0.5	0
Coleslaw	3	91	119	1.5	13.3	1	6.6	1.0	5
Original Recipe Chicken									
Wing	2	55	178	12.2	6.0	0	11.7	3.0	64
Breast	4	115	283	27.5	8.8	0	15.3	3.8	93
Drumstick	2	57	146	13.1	4.2	0	8.5	2.2	67
Thigh	4	104	294	17.9	11.1	1	19.7	5.3	123
Extra Crispy Chicken									
Wing	2	65	254	12.4	9.3	0	18.6	4.0	67
Breast	5	135	342	33.0	11.7	1	19.7	4.8	114
Drumstick	2	69	204	13.6	6.1	0	13.9	3.4	71
Thigh	4	119	406	20.0	14.4	1	29.8	7.7	129
Restaurant: Long John Silver's Seafood Shoppe									
3-pc Fish Lt/Paprika (Baked)	5	134	120	28.0	1.0	0	1.0	0.4	110
3-pc Fish/Lemon Crumb (Baked)	5	141	150	29.0	4.0	0	1.0	0.4	110

44

Food Name	Oz	Gm	KCAL Gm	PROT Gm	CARB Gm	FIBD Gm	FAT Gm	SAFA Gm	CHOL Mg
3-pc Fish/Scampi Sauce (Baked)	5	148	170	28.0	2.0	0	5.0	2.9	110
Shrimp/Scampi Sauce (Baked)	5	148	120	15.0	2.0	0	5.0	3.2	205
Chicken Light/Herbs (Baked)	4	117	140	25.0	1.0	0	4.0	1.2	70
Restaurant: McDonald's									
Egg McMuffin	5	138	290	18.2	28.1	1	11.2	3.8	226
Hotcakes/Butter/Syrup	6	176	410	8.2	74.4	2	9.2	3.7	21
Scrambled Eggs	4	100	140	12.4	1.2	0	9.8	3.3	399
Pork Sausage	2	48	180	8.4	0.0	0	16.3	5.9	48
English Muffin/Butter	2	59	170	5.4	26.7	1	4.6	2.4	9
Hashbrown Potatoes	2	53	130	1.4	14.9	2	7.3	3.2	9
Biscuit/Biscuit Spread	3	75	260	4.6	31.9	1	12.7	3.4	1
Biscuit/Sausage	4	123	440	13.0	31.9	1	29.0	9.3	49
Biscuit/Sausage/Egg	6	180	520	19.9	32.6	1	34.5	11.2	275
Biscuit/Bacon/Egg/Cheese	6	156	440	17.5	33.3	1	26.4	8.2	253
Sausage McMuffin	6	117	370	16.5	27.3	1	21.9	7.8	64
Sausage McMuffin/Cheese	6	167	440	22.6	27.9	1	26.8	9.5	263
Apple Danish	4	115	390	5.8	51.2	2	17.9	3.5	25
Iced Cheese Danish	4	110	390	7.4	42.3	1	21.8	6.0	47
Cinnamon Raisin Danish	4	110	440	6.4	57.5	2	21.0	4.2	34
Raspberry Danish	4	117	410	6.1	61.5	2	15.9	3.1	26
Apple Bran Muffin	3	85	190	5.0	46.0	2	0.0	0.0	0
Blueberry Muffin	3	85	170	3.0	40.0	1	0.0	0.0	0

Food Name	Oz	Gm	KCAL Gm	PROT Gm	CARB Gm	FIBD Gm	FAT Gm	SAFA Gm	CHOL Mg
Chicken McNuggets	4	113	290	19.0	16.5	1	16.3	4.1	65
Hamburger	4	102	260	12.3	30.6	1	9.5	3.6	37
Cheeseburger	4	116	310	15.0	31.2	1	13.8	5.2	53
McLean Deluxe	7	203	310	20.0	34.0	2	10.0	4.6	37
Quarter Pounder	6	166	410	23.1	34.0	1	20.7	8.1	86
Quarter Pounder/Cheese	7	194	520	28.5	35.1	1	29.2	11.2	118
Big Mac	8	215	560	25.2	42.5	1	32.4	10.1	103
Filet-O-Fish	5	142	440	13.8	37.9	1	26.1	5.2	50
McD.L.T.	8	234	580	26.3	36.0	2	36.8	11.5	109
McChicken	7	190	490	19.2	39.8	1	28.6	5.4	43
Chef Salad	10	283	230	20.5	7.5	2	13.3	5.9	128
Garden Salad	8	213	110	7.1	6.2	2	6.6	2.9	83
Chicken Salad Oriental	9	244	140	23.1	5.0	2.	3.4	0.9	78
Side Salad	4	115	60	3.7	3.3	1	3.3	1.5	41
French Fries, Small	2	68	220	3.1	25.6	2	12.0	5.1	9
French Fries, Medium	3	97	320	4.4	36.3	3	17.1	7.2	12
French Fries, Large	4	122	400	5.6	45.9	3	21.6	9.1	16
Apple Pie	3	83	260	2.2	30.0	2	14.8	4.8	6
Vanilla Lowfat Milk Shake	11	293	290	10.8	60.0	0	1.3	0.6	10
Chocolate Lowfat Milk Shake	11	293	320	11.0	66.0	1	1.7	0.8	10
Strawberry Lowfat Milk Shake	11	293	320	10.7	67.0	0	1.3	0.6	10
McDonaldland Cookies	2	56	290	4.2	47.1	1	9.2	1.8	0
Chocolaty Chip Cookies	2	56	330	4.2	41.9	0	15.6	5.0	4

46

Food Name	Oz	Gm	KCAL Gm	PROT Gm	CARB Gm	FIBD Gm	FAT Gm	SAFA Gm	CHOL Mg
Restaurant: Pizza Hut									
Pan Pizza, 2 slices									
Cheese	7	205	492	30.0	57.0	5	18.0	9.3	34
Pepperoni	8	211	540	29.0	62.0	5	22.0	10.9	42
Supreme	9	255	589	32.0	53.0	7	30.0	11.6	48
Super Supreme	9	257	563	33.0	53.0	6	26.0	11.1	55
Thin 'n Crispy Pizza, 2 slices									
Cheese	5	148	398	28.0	37.0	4	17.0	10.2	33
Pepperoni	5	146	413	26.0	20.0	4	20.0	8.9	46
Supreme	7	200	459	28.0	41.0	5	22.0	9.0	42
Super Supreme	7	203	463	29.0	44.0	5	21.0	9.3	56
Hand-Tossed Pizza, 2 slices									
Cheese	8	220	518	34.0	55.0	7	20.0	9.9	55
Pepperoni	7	197	500	28.0	50.0	6	23.0	10.2	50
Supreme	8	239	540	32.0	50.0	7	26.0	11.1	55
Super Supreme	9	243	556	33.0	54.0	7	25.0	11.4	54
Personal Pan Pizza, 1 pizza									
Pepperoni	9	256	675	37.0	76.0	8	29.0	13.7	53
Supreme	9	264	647	33.0	76.0	9	28.0	13.2	49
Restaurant: Taco Bell									
Bean Burrito/Red Sauce	7	191	356	13.1	54.4	5	10.2	2.9	9
Beef Burrito/Red Sauce	7	191	403	22.5	39.1	3	17.3	7.4	57
Burrito Supreme/Red Sauce	9	241	413	18.0	46.6	4	17.6	7.7	33
Dble Beef Burrito Supreme Red Sauce	9	255	457	23.7	41.7	-	21.8	10.1	57

Food Name	Oz Gm	KCAL Gm	PROT Gm	CARB Gm	FIBD Gm	FAT Gm	SAFA Gm	CHOL Mg
Tostada/Red Sauce	6	156	243	9.5	26.6	6	11.1	4.1	16
Enchirito/Red Sauce	8	213	382	19.8	30.9	4	19.7	9.3	54
Cinnamon Crispas	2	47	259	2.7	27.5	2	15.3	3.7	1
Pintos & Cheese/Red Sauce	5	128	191	9.0	19.0	4	8.7	3.6	16
Nachos	4	106	346	7.5	37.5	4	18.5	5.7	9
Nachos Bellgrande	10	287	649	21.6	60.6	7	35.3	12.3	36
Taco	28	778	183	10.3	11.0	1	10.8	4.6	32
Taco Bellgrande	6	163	355	18.3	17.7	2	23.1	11.0	56
Taco Light	6	170	410	19.0	18.1	2	28.8	11.6	56
Soft Taco	3	92	228	11.8	17.9	1	11.9	5.4	32
Soft Taco Supreme	4	124	275	12.6	19.1	1	16.3	8.1	32
Taco Salad/Salsa	21	595	941	36.0	63.1	10	61.3	18.7	80
Taco Salad/Salsa w/o Shell	19	530	520	30.6	30.0	6	31.4	14.4	80
Taco Salad without Shell	19	530	520	29.5	26.3	6	31.3	14.4	80
Mexican Pizza	8	223	575	21.3	39.7	6	36.8	11.4	52
Taco Sauce	<1	<1	2	0.1	0.4	0	0.0	0.0	0
Hot Taco Sauce	<1	<1	3	0.1	0.3	0	0.1	0.0	0
Jalapeno Peppers	5	100	20	1.0	4.0	1	0.2	0.1	0
Steak Fajita	5	135	234	14.6	19.5	1	10.9	4.8	14
Chicken Fajita	5	135	226	13.6	19.8	1	10.2	3.7	44
Sour Cream	1	21	46	0.6	0.9	0	4.4	2.7	16
Pico De Gallo	1	28	8	0.3	1.1	0	0.2	0.0	1
Guacamole	4	21	34	0.4	3.0	1	2.3	0.4	0
Meximelt	4	106	266	12.9	18.7	1	15.4	7.9	38

Food Name	Oz	Gm	KCAL Gm	PROT Gm	CARB Gm	FIBD Gm	FAT Gm	SAFA Gm	CHOL Mg
Restaurant: Wendy's Old Fashioned Hamburgers									
Junior Hamburger	3	104	260	15.0	32.0	1	9.0	3.3	35
Junior Cheeseburger	3	116	300	18.0	33.0	1	13.0	6.4	35
Small Hamburger	4	111	260	15.0	33.0	1	9.0	3.4	34
Small Cheeseburger	4	125	310	18.0	33.0	1	13.0	7.2	34
Chicken Sandwich	8	219	430	26.0	41.0	2	19.0	4.6	60
Big Classic/Cheese	10	295	640	30.0	46.0	4	38.0	12.5	100
Plain Single	4	126	340	24.0	30.0	1	15.0	6.4	65
Single/Everything	8	210	420	25.0	35.0	1	21.0	5.6	70
Plain Single/Cheese	5	137	410	25.0	29.0	1	22.0	10.6	80
Garden Salad (Take-Out)	10	227	102	7.0	9.0	4	5.0	2.3	0
Chef Salad (Take-Out)	12	331	180	15.0	10.0	4	9.0	5.2	120
New Chili	9	256	220	21.0	23.0	7	7.0	2.9	45
Taco Salad	28	791	660	40.0	46.0	9	37.0	15.9	35
French Fries, Small	3	91	240	3.0	33.0	2	12.0	4.6	15
Restaurant: White Castle									
Hamburger	2	58	161	5.9	15.4	2	7.9	2.8	18
Cheeseburger	2	65	200	7.8	15.5	3	11.2	4.9	28
Fish Sandwich w/o	2	59	155	5.8	20.9	1	5.0	1.2	8
Tartar Sauce									
Sausage/Egg Sandwich	3	96	322	12.6	16.1	3	22.0	6.4	151
Sausage Sandwich	2	49	196	6.7	13.3	2	12.3	3.7	22
Chicken Sandwich	2	64	186	8.0	20.5	2	7.5	1.6	1.9
French Fries	3	97	301	2.5	37.7	5	14.7	2.3	0
Onion Rings	2	63	246	2.9	26.6	3	13.4	2.1	0

ENERGY COSTS OF
VARIOUS ACTIVITIES

Activity	Body Weight		
	120 Pounds (54 Kilograms) Kcal/Hour	150 Pounds (68 Kilograms) Kcal/Hour	180 Pounds (82 Kilograms) Kcal/Hour
Aerobics—heavy	435	544	653
Aerobics—light	163	204	244
Aerobics—medium	272	340	408
Back-packing	489	612	734
Badminton	277	346	416
Ballroom dancing	166	208	249
Basketball—vigorous	544	680	816
Bicycling (5.5 MPH)	163	204	244
Billiards	108	136	163
Bowling	212	265	318
Calisthenics—heavy	435	544	653
Calisthenics—light	217	272	326
Canoeing (2.5 MPH)	179	224	269
Carpentry—general	272	340	408
Circuit training	604	755	906
Cleaning (F)	202	253	303
Cleaning (M)	189	236	284
Climbing (100 FT/HR)	391	489	587
Cooking (F)	146	183	220
Cooking (M)	156	195	235
Cycling (13 MPH)	527	659	791
Disco dancing	326	408	489
Ditch digging—hand	315	394	473
Dressing/showering	85	106	128
Driving	93	117	140
Eating (sitting)	75	93	112

Activity	Body Weight		
	120 Pounds (54 Kilograms) Kcal/Hour	150 Pounds (68 Kilograms) Kcal/Hour	180 Pounds (82 Kilograms) Kcal/Hour
Fencing	239	299	359
Food shopping (F)	202	253	303
Food shopping (M)	189	236	284
Football—touch	380	476	571
Gardening	174	217	261
Gardening—digging	411	514	617
Gardening—raking	176	220	264
Golf	195	244	293
Horseback riding—trotting	277	346	416
Housework—cleaning	217	272	326
Ice skating (10 MPH)	315	394	473
Jazzercize—heavy	435	544	653
Jazzercize—light	163	204	244
Jazzercize—medium	272	340	408
Jogging—medium	489	612	734
Jogging—slow	380	476	571
Judo	636	795	955
Lawn mowing (hand)	212	265	318
Lawn mowing (power)	195	244	293
Lying—at ease	71	89	107
Piano playing	130	163	195
Racquetball—social	435	544	653
Roller skating	277	346	416
Rowboating (2.5 MPH)	239	299	369

Activity	Body Weight		
	120 Pounds (54 Kilograms) Kcal/Hour	150 Pounds (68 Kilograms) Kcal/Hour	180 Pounds (82 Kilograms) Kcal/Hour
Running or jogging (10 MPH)	718	897	1077
Scull rowing (race)	669	836	1004
Sewing—hand	104	130	156
Shuffleboard/skeet	163	204	244
Sitting quietly	68	85	102
Skiing (10 MPH)	478	598	718
Sleeping	64	80	97
Square dancing	277	346	416
Squash or handball	478	598	718
Swimming (.25 MPH)	239	299	359
Table tennis	282	353	424
Tennis	331	414	497
Volleyball	277	346	416
Walking (2.5 MPH)	163	204	244
Walking (3.75 MPH)	239	299	359
Water skiing	380	476	571
Weight lifting—heavy	489	612	734
Weight lifting—light	217	272	326
Window cleaning (F)	192	240	288
Window cleaning (M)	189	236	284
Woodchopping/sawing	315	394	473
Writing (sitting)	94	118	142

DIET RECORD FORMS

Time	Min Spent Eating	Activity While Eating	Reason for Eating Place of Eating	Food & Quantity

Time	Min Spent Eating	Activity While Eating	Reason for Eating Place of Eating	Food & Quantity

Time	Min Spent Eating	Activity While Eating	Reason for Eating Place of Eating	Food & Quantity

Time	Min Spent Eating	Activity While Eating	Reason for Eating / Place of Eating	Food & Quantity

Time	Min Spent Eating	Activity While Eating	Reason for Eating Place of Eating	Food & Quantity

Time	Min Spent Eating	Activity While Eating	Reason for Eating Place of Eating	Food & Quantity

Time	Min Spent Eating	Activity While Eating	Reason for Eating Place of Eating	Food & Quantity